The Ultimate
DIABETIC
COOKBOOK
FOR BEGINNERS

Easy and Healthy Low-carb Recipes Book for
Type 2 Diabetes Newly Diagnosed to Live Better
(21 Days Meal Plan Included)

JAMIE PRESS

Table of Content

Introduction...1

Chapter 1: The Basics of Type 2
Diabetes..3
The Trend of Diabetes 3
What Causes Type-2 Diabetes? 3
Differences Between Type-1 and Type-2
Diabetes..4
Don't Worry When You Have Prediabetes   4
Treatment for Diabetes...........................5

Chapter 2: Diabetes and Nutrition 6
Other Essential Nutrients.......................7
Counting Macronutrients.......................7
Watch What You Eat................................8

Chapter 3: A Fresh Start 10
Plan Your Plate...................................... 10
Changing Your Kitchen 11
Special Occasions and Other Challenges...12

Chapter 4: 21-Day Meal Plan 13

Chapter 5 Breakfast 15
Simple Grain-Free Biscuits 15
Brussels Sprout with Fried Eggs............. 15
Carrot and Oat Pancakes 16
Savory Breakfast Egg Bites 16
Vanilla Coconut Pancakes...................... 17
Cheesy Spinach and Egg Casserole 17
Scrumptious Orange Muffins 18
Easy Turkey Breakfast Patties................ 18
Pecan-Oatmeal Pancakes 19
Peanut Butter and Berry Oatmeal 19
Quick Breakfast Yogurt Sundae.............. 20

Chapter 6 Appetizers................................20
Aromatic Toasted Pumpkin Seeds........... 20
Bacon-Wrapped Shrimps 21
Cheesy Broccoli Bites 21
Easy Caprese Skewers 22
Grilled Tofu with Sesame Seeds............. 22
Kale Chips 23
Simple Deviled Eggs 23

Chapter 7 Vegetable Sides.......................24
Sautéed Collard Greens and Cabbage......24
Roasted Delicata Squash with Thyme 24
Roasted Asparagus and Red Peppers 25
Tarragon Spring Peas 25
Butter-Orange Yams 26
Roasted Tomato Brussels Sprouts 26
Simple Sautéed Greens 27
Garlicky Mushrooms.............................. 27
Sesame Bok Choy with Almonds 28
Lime Asparagus with Cashews............... 28

Chapter 8 Meatless Mains 29
Roasted Tomato and Bell Pepper Soup.....29
Sautéed Zucchini and Tomatoes 29
Roasted Brussels Sprouts with Wild Rice
Bowl..30
Cheesy Mushroom and Pesto Flatbreads...30
Butternut Noodles With Mushroom Sauce.31
Homemade Vegetable Chili 31
Wilted Dandelion Greens with Sweet Onion
....32
Collard Greens with Tomato 32
Cheesy Summer Squash and Quinoa
Casserole 33
Creamy Macaroni and Cheese 33
Spaghetti Puttanesca 34

Chapter 9 Beans, Grains, and Legumes....34

Crispy Cowboy Black Bean Fritters 34
Macaroni and Vegetable Pie................... 35
Dandelion and Beet Greens 35
Black Bean and Tomato Soup with Lime Yogurt...36
Classic Texas Caviar............................ 36
Brown Rice with Carrot, and Scrambled Egg 37
Black Bean, Corn, and Chicken Soup 37
Wild Rice and Cranberries Salad.............38
Red Kidney Beans with Tomatoes 39

Chapter 10 Fish and Seafood Mains 39

Marinated Grilled Salmon with Lemongrass ..
....39
Broiled Teriyaki Salmon 40
Roasted Vegetable and Chicken Tortillas...40
Tartar Tuna Patties............................. 41
Lemon Parsley White Fish Fillets 41
Fresh Rosemary Trout 42
Butter-Lemon Grilled Cod on Asparagus...42
Cioppino (Seafood and Tomato Stew) 43
Grilled Shrimp Skewers with Yogurt 43
Cilantro Lime Shrimp 44
Panko Coconut Shrimp 44
Shrimp Coleslaw................................. 45

Chapter 11 Poultry Mains 45

Herbed Chicken and Artichoke Hearts...... 45
Citrus Chicken Thighs.......................... 46
Creamy and Aromatic Chicken................ 46
Creamy and Cheesy Chicken Chile Casserole
....47
Roasted Chicken with Root Vegetables.....48
Ritzy Jerked Chicken Breasts.................. 49
Blackened Spatchcock with Lime Aioli...... 49
Turkey Meatball and Vegetable Kabobs 50
Chicken with Carrot, and Kale 51

Chapter 12 Pork, Beef, and Lamb Mains....52

Sumptuous Lamb and Pomegranate Salad52
Chipotle Chili Pork 53
Pork Diane.. 53
Pork Souvlakia with Tzatziki Sauce.......... 54
Beef, Tomato, and Pepper Tortillas 54
Classic Stroganoff................................ 55
Easy Lime Lamb Cutlets 55
Spinach, Pear, and Walnut Salad............. 56
Ritzy Beef Stew................................... 56
Slow Cooked Beef and Vegetables Roast...57

Chapter 13 Soups, Salads, and Sandwiches...57

Chicken and Zoodle Soup 57
Ritzy Calabaza Squash Soup 58
Simple Buttercup Squash Soup............... 58
Turkey, Barley and Vegetable Stock......... 59
Shrimp and Cherry Tomato Salad............ 59
Citrus Pork Tenderloin 60
Mexican Turkey Sliders 60
Cheesy Vegetable and Hummus Pitas 61
Seafood, Mango, and Avocado Salad 61

Chapter 14 Desserts 62

Crispy Apple Chips............................... 62
Date and Almond Balls with Seeds 62
Apple Cinnamon Chimichanga 63
Chia and Raspberry Pudding 63
Easy Banana Mug Cake 64
Pumpkin and Raspberry Muffins.............. 64

Chapter 15 Staples.................................65

Avocado Cilantro Dressing 65
Lemon Tahini Dressing with Honey.......... 65
Red Pepper and Chickpea Spread............ 66
Mayo Ketchup Sauce 66
Spicy Asian Dipping Sauce 67
Easy Thai Peanut Sauce........................ 67
Chimichurri.. 68
Appendix 1: Measurement conversion Chart 69
Appendix 2: Recipes Index 70

Introduction

There wasn't a time in my life that I don't remember indulging in food. From the time that I was a little tot, my tongue had a serious appetite for different tastes, flavors, and textures. It was an instant love affair and food has been my partner ever since.

You couldn't stop me from being in the kitchen if you tried. I was 8 years old when I first started tinkering away with different flavors—always with the help of my parents, of course. I loved the way a roux sauce complemented crunchy vegetables or the béchamel that lay on top of the perfect lasagna. When I say I loved food, I really mean it. Unfortunately, like with all things in life, I had a few roadblocks ahead of me that would make me question my relationship with food.

When I was 37 years old, I got what I thought was the most soul-crushing news. I still remember the day like it was yesterday. It's a memory I don't think I'll ever lose.

I had gone to see my doctor because my vision had gone blurry at certain times in the day, and my energy levels were not what they once were. I was tired all the time! I remember I stared at my hands, as I waited for the doctor to come back with my blood work, because they were numb all over. I imagined a hundred different scenarios, but as that door opened and my doctor shuffled back in, I never expected him to tell me, "You are diabetic."

It sounds like I'm joking, but my world shattered. I didn't know much about being diabetic then, but I knew that diabetics had to follow a different set of diet rules. All of a sudden the homemade ice-creams, chocolate chip cookies, and red velvet cakes that I loved to make and indulge in seemed far out of my reach. I thought I would have to give up my love affair with food. I thought I'd never be allowed to eat a rich dessert again for fear of angering the diabetic Gods out there.

I stood at the edge of the precipice that I was ready to fall down from. This seemed impossible!

That is until I pulled my boots up and decided that I needed to tackle this diagnosis with the same zest I had tackled my love for food, before my diagnosis. It wasn't going to be easy. I didn't know anyone in my life who was diabetic, I was the first. So, I had to do a lot of the legwork on my own. I mean, how did I even know what to eat and how to eat? What was my body doing to it itself? There were a ton of unanswered questions in my life.

I decided to dedicate the next few years of my life to learning and embracing a diabetic lifestyle. I was determined to rebuild my relationship with food. I didn't want to miss out on the flavors of life simply because I was diabetic. I had to find other ways to do this. So, that's exactly what I did.

Today, I stand up tall and proud and I can say that I have restored my relationship with food. I never ever feel like I'm missing out because I know that my food tastes as delicious as the food that I was eating before I got my diagnosis. In fact, my diabetic diagnosis opened up an entirely new world in the kitchen for me. It felt almost selfish to keep all this knowledge—and tasty food—to myself.

In this cookbook, I've decided to impart all the recipes, tips, and information that I've learned throughout the years. If you're struggling and pulling your hair out, wondering how you're going to cope with a restricted diet, relax. I was there once too and stress does nothing more than push your blood pressure up.

Now, I no longer stress about what I'm going to eat. I'm even calm when I go out to restaurants with friends. I no longer shy away from girls' nights out. Instead, I embrace them because I've taken my health and diet into my own hands.

As you read this book, you'll gain the confidence that you need to take your health into your own hands. As we explore chapter one, you'll get a better understanding of what type-2 diabetes is and how it affects your body. There's a lot of information regarding your own health that you might be too scared to ask your own doctor. I answer all those burning questions for you.

In chapter two, our focus shifts from what diabetes is to how it relates to nutrition. It's important to know about those macronutrients that you're putting in your body. Confused? Don't worry, you'll understand it all at the end of this chapter.

Chapter three will tie everything together when it comes to watching what and how you eat, as well as prepping your kitchen. There will inevitably be changes that you need to make in your lifestyle. This might mean you need a few more kitchen tools, and you'll also have to toss out some unhealthy kitchen habits. We cover it all here.

As you get more comfortable with being a type-2 diabetic and the food changes that come with that, you'll want to brave going out to eat. After all, being a diabetic doesn't mean you have to become a hermit. This book arms you with the tools you'll need to handle those situations when you're out and about.

Of course, I can't forget those taste enriching recipes that this cookbook I've promised you in the title! It's not enough to know what diabetes is and what to eat. I am going to arm you with some easy, delicious recipes that will set your taste buds alight. I'm talking about all that flavor and zest that you thought you had to miss out on. The recipes I've chosen have been successfully tried out, and there's something for more than one type of eater in here.

My goal is that you are empowered with your diagnosis to take control of it with this guide. I know that healthy and tasty eating is possible. Being a diabetic hasn't stopped me from indulging in all of life's flavors, and it shouldn't stop you either.

Happy indulging!

Chapter 1: The Basics of Type 2 Diabetes

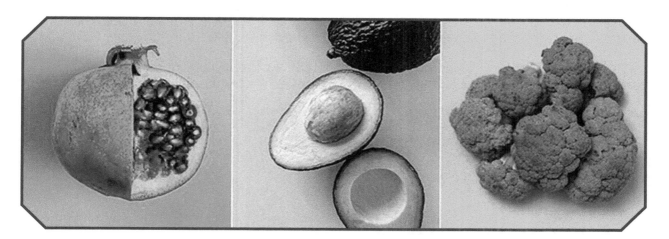

The Trend of Diabetes

Diabetes has emerged as one common and chronic disease around the world. In the United States, along about 23.1 million people have been diagnosed with Diabetes, which has cost about $245 billion annually. The center for disease control has recently calculated that more people are entering into this loop, and their estimates suggest the figure to be 7.2 million, which are yet to be diagnosed with Diabetes. Whereas 84.1 million adults in the US are suffering from prediabetes. The prevalence of Diabetes is common among minorities and increases with rates of obesity and overweight in the country. Those who are already suffering from Diabetes are at a higher risk of heart stroke, other heart diseases, depression, pain, hypertension, functional disabilities, and polypharmacy. The condition is also claimed to be the leading cause of some cases of blindness and renal failure. There are several more figures to support that the threats of Diabetes are ever-increasing now more than ever. This gradual rise in the prevalence of the diseases suggests one thing that the factors causing the diseases are also rising or that they are not adequately dealt with.

What Causes Type-2 Diabetes?

Type-2 diabetes means that your body's cells fail to communicate and process insulin. This means that there can be an abnormally large build-up on insulin if left uncontrolled. When diabetes gets to a late-stage you might even find that your body isn't able to produce enough insulin for your needs.

There isn't only one cause or reason for diabetes, but many. Your genes and family history are important when it comes to diabetes. If you have a family member that has type-2 diabetes than you are more than likely predisposed to get it as well.

Your age also plays a role. As you age, your risk goes up with you. Men and women who are over 45 years of age are more likely to be diagnosed with diabetes.

Obesity and a poor diet are leading factors in diabetic diagnoses. Bear in mind that having a poor diet doesn't always correlate to obesity. If you eat a diet full of simple carbohydrates or sugars, your body builds up an insulin resistance—which is what causes type-2 diabetes.

Differences Between Type-1 and Type-2 Diabetes

There are fundamental differences between type-1 and type-2 diabetes. Those who are type-1 don't produce insulin at all. Their immune systems attack the healthy cells that the pancreas needs to produce insulin. This leaves the person unable to produce any insulin.

In type-2 diabetes, the person is insulin resistant. As the disease progresses their pancreas might stop producing insulin as well, however, we try to avoid this stage.

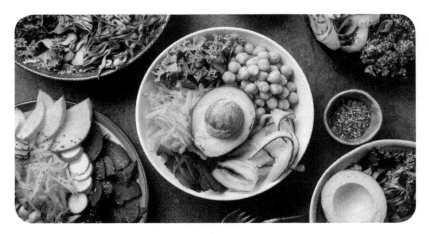

Don't Worry When You Have Prediabetes

Have you ever heard of the term prediabetic? Simply put, those who are prediabetic have high blood sugar levels, yet they aren't necessarily diabetic yet. Most people who end up with a type-2 diabetes diagnosis will have had prediabetes. The issue is because it rarely shows symptoms, it's hard to catch.

Here's the kicker. If you can catch your diabetes when you're in the prediabetic stage, you're one step ahead of solving your health issues. You can prevent a type-2 diabetic diagnosis if you take control of your health.

In order to prevent diabetes, you need to make sure that you:

◆ *Eat a balanced diet, reducing simple carbs*
◆ *Exercise*
◆ *Cut down and stop smoking*

Treatment for Diabetes

There are several different treatment options for diabetes. You can use insulin medications, non-insulin medications, weight loss, and diet changes in order to treat your diabetes.

Checking your blood sugar level is going to become a big part of your day if it hasn't already. In order to get a reading using your blood glucose meter, you need to make sure that you've washed your hands. Then, prick yourself on the side of your finger. You only need a drop of blood. Let the test strip that's attached to your device touch the blood and wait for your reading.

As a diabetic, you're going to learn a lot about your glycemic index and load. The glycemic index is really important because it tells you how certain foods will affect your blood sugar level. What does this mean for you? Well, we give glucose (or pure sugar) a value of 100. If the food's GI is less than 100 then it will impact your blood sugar levels less.

The Glycemic Load is an equation you can use that calculates the GI of a planned portion size. This lets you know if you're eating too much or too little of that type of food. Eating a lot of low GI food can still be an overabundance if you're eating more than you should.

Exercise is an important part of keeping your body healthy and lowering your risk of getting type-2 diabetes. It's a great way to manage your diabetes if you've already been living with it for a while. Don't forget to make exercise a part of your daily routine, even if it is only a 30-minute walk every day.

Being a type-2 diabetic can take a toll on someone mentally. I suggest that you reach out to support groups. Your doctor should have resources for groups that meet in person, but you can also reach out through social media. If you find that you need to speak to a counselor, don't be shy. It's a huge transition to make in your life and sometimes you need a little extra help.

Chapter 2: Diabetes and Nutrition

If you've never heard of macronutrients, get ready to have your world opened. Eating right and eating healthy is about more than meeting a certain caloric intake per day. It's also about understanding what group your calories come from and how many you need.

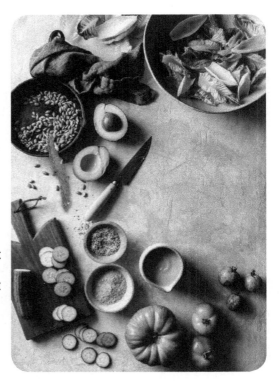

I know that this can be one of the more frustrating aspects to figure out, but once you've got it down you'll wonder why you never counted your macronutrients before.

Your macros include carbohydrates, protein, and fats.

Let's start with carbohydrates. It's first important to note that not all carbohydrates are created equal. You have complex carbs and simple carbs. A complex carbohydrate will take longer for your body to break down. Green vegetables and fibrous fruits are good examples of complex carbs. A simple carb will be processed by your body much faster, like sugary drinks and syrups, bread and pasta.

Complex carbs will give you a longer source of energy, where simple carbs give your body a short burst of energy and a blood sugar level spike. So, it's important to know what your body needs when you're eating.

Protein is necessary for building your muscles up. You can get your protein either from plant-based sources or animal-based sources. The important thing is that protein is needed for diabetics, so if you love to eat your meat, this means you don't have to give that up.

I know that fat is a dreaded word and many people try to stay away from eating too much of it, however, it's also an important macronutrient. You can have saturated fats, unsaturated fats, and trans fat. As a diabetic, you're going to want to stick with the unsaturated fats.

Unsaturated fats can be found in nuts, fish, avocados, and olive oil. These fats help lower your levels of bad cholesterol and control your levels of blood sugar. They have also been known to lower blood pressure.

Saturated fats are often found in meats and dairy products. These fats are not healthy for you or your arteries. You shouldn't eat more than 15 grams of saturated fats a day. You can look at 15 grams as equivalent to one cup of your favorite ice cream.

Trans fats are human-made fats - aka artificial. They'll be found in your store-bought cakes and cookies. These are the types of fats that you want to avoid point-blank. They raise your levels of bad cholesterol and can lead to serious complications if consumed too much.

Every person, and every body, is different. This means that your needs for macronutrients might look different from mine. While the American Diabetes Association does have a recommended diabetic macronutrient intake, it's important to remember that you might have to adjust these values to your body's needs.

Traditionally, a diabetic should plan out their macronutrients in these amounts:

* *55-65% carbohydrates, with the vast majority of those being complex (fruits and vegetables)*
* *10-20% of proteins*
* *30% or less of fats.*

Other Essential Nutrients

Your macronutrients are important, however, you still need other nutrients to make your health whole. When you're eating, make sure that your foods have vitamin D, magnesium, and sodium in them.

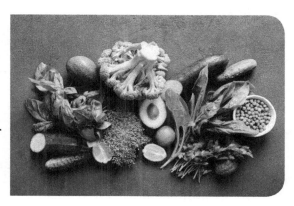

Because magnesium levels are generally lower in people with diabetes, it's important that, either as a supplement or in the foods you're eating, you get enough magnesium to replace what you are losing.

Vitamin D is crucial as it boosts your insulin sensitivity. Getting enough sun or taking a supplement can help you regulate your blood sugar levels.

While sodium is good for you, it needs to be consumed in moderation. You should try to limit your salt intake to no more than one teaspoon per day. This helps with your blood pressure.

As you go through your dietary changes, you'll naturally learn a lot. It's a necessary adjustment, but it doesn't have to be a bad one. When you stick to those good unsaturated fats and you're conscious of where you get your macronutrients from, you'll find that taking care of your body isn't as daunting as it first seemed. You'll learn so much more about yourself.

Counting Macronutrients

When we talk about macronutrients, we mean your carbohydrates, proteins, and fats. You're probably already used to some form of counting calories already—especially if you've tried one of the many diets out there. This is simply taking it one step up from calorie counting.

* *One gram of carbohydrates is equal to 4 calories.*
* *One gram of fat is equal to 9 calories.*
* *One gram of protein is equal to 4 calories.*

Do you see where this ties into your calorie counting yet?

You can use the traditional numbers given above to count your macronutrients, or you can figure out your own specific needs by finding out what your resting energy expenditure and non-resting energy expenditure are.

When you add your REE and your NREE together you get the total calories that you burn every day. There are dozens of online calculators that you can use to figure this out. You simply need to search for them, and they'll pop up. Most of them take less than thirty seconds to give you your results.

Once you know your macronutrient needs, you can start tracking them. This can be done with a phone app, a journal you keep, or with any other method that is best suited to your lifestyle.

So, how do you count the macronutrients once you have all this information?

Let's take our values above. This diet needs 60% carbs, 15% proteins, and 25% fats. I need to consume 1800 calories a day.

So, for my carbs, I'll find out what 60% of 1800 calories is. This leaves me with 1080 calories of carbs to consume every day.

1080 calories divided by 4 grams of carbs gives me 270 grams. So, every day, my macronutrient goal for carbohydrates will be no more than 270 grams. You use this same method for proteins and fats to easily find out how many grams of each you should be eating.

When you buy food, this information should be available to you on the back of the nutritional information packet. Some apps have barcode scanners that take the guesswork out of this and automatically gives you the macronutrient breakdown of the food you're buying.

Watch What You Eat

The diabetic diet is not high restrictive; it just eliminates the food from the menu, which can lead to high levels of blood glucose levels, even in the absence of insulin. To do so, the following ingredients are suitable to consume on a diabetic diet:

◆ Vegetables: both starchy and non-starchy including broccoli, carrots, greens, peppers, and tomatoes, potatoes, corn, and green peas

◆ Fruits—like berries, melon, oranges, apples, pears, peach, apricots and grapes

◆ Grains—like whole grains: cornmeal, wheat, brown rice, oats, barley, and quinoa

◆ Dried beans and peas, like chickpeas and split peas

◆ Seafood and fish, like salmon, tuna, sardines, shrimp
◆ Lean meat
◆ Chicken or turkey
◆ Eggs
◆ Nuts and peanuts
◆ Fat-free plain Yogurt
◆ Low-fat or skim milk
◆ Low-fat Cheese
◆ Unsaturated plant-based oils
◆ Avocado

> **Whereas food which can be damaging for diabetic patients, including the following items:**
>
> ◈ *Fried foods and foods high in trans-fat and saturated fats*
> ◈ *Foods high in salt also called sodium*
> ◈ *Sweets, like baked goods, candy, and ice cream*

Beverages with sugars, like regular soda, juice, and energy drinks

You don't have to give up those foods you love when you become a diabetic. You simply need to modify them to your body's needs and watch your portions. In fact, portion control is one of the biggest aspects of any type of diet.

When you control the size of your portions, you eat less. Generally, people eat twice as much as they need to because they have a big plate, and they think filling it is the way to go.

Try this fun activity with your family. Put on a blindfold and have someone put a plate of food in front of you. Eat until you feel full—not stuffed, but full. Then take the blindfold off and see how much you ate. I promise you'll probably be surprised at how little you've eaten from the plate.

I suggest using smaller plates. This helps you put less food on your plate, and you'll still feel full afterward.

Another tip is to drink a glass of water at the start of your meal. This way you'll feel fuller and you won't overindulge during the meal.

As a diabetic, you need to be cautious when you drink alcohol. Alcohol heightens your blood sugar levels and leaves you susceptible to hypoglycemia. If your diabetes is well managed, then I suggest you drink your alcohol before, during, or right after eating. Don't overindulge in alcohol, because this can still have negative effects on you.

Have you ever heard of sugar alcohol? It's simply a sweetener that is normally found in foods that contain low-fat or diet advertising. You might have heard it called other names such as xylitol, glycerin, or isomalt.

It has less of an effect on your blood sugar levels, but you should still watch how much of it you eat. It's safer for diabetics to consume sugar alcohols but don't go overboard with it.

Chapter 3: A Fresh Start

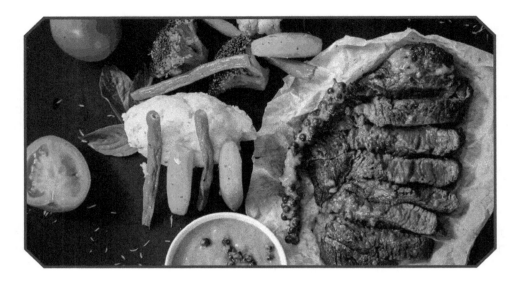

Plan Your Plate

The diabetic menu should aspire to achieve a balance of carbohydrates and nutrients, such as proteins and healthy fats. This is essential for proper diabetes management and also to ensure that the meals are satisfying.

About half of your meal should be non-starchy vegetables. One portion should be proteins, while the remaining portion should be grains or starch.

Remember the following:

➊ 20% to 25% of the calories should be from protein. Remember, lean meats like beef and chicken are better.

➋ 25% to 30% of the calories must be from fat. Stay away or limit the intake of saturated and trans fats.

➌ 50% to 60% of the calories must be from carbohydrates. You must eat plenty of orange and green vegetables every day, such as broccoli and carrots. Opt for brown rice that is vitamin-rich or sweet potatoes, while avoiding regular potatoes or white rice.

Maintain a food diary for the first few days so that you know what you like and dislike. Keep it detailed. You can then modify your food menu accordingly while maintaining the basic diabetes food principles.

But remember, some modifications might be necessary, especially if you have other goals, like for instance, to lose weight. Calorie counting will then be also needed. Again, if you want to build muscles, then you will have to take lower fat and increase the percentage of carbohydrates.

Changing Your Kitchen

Inevitably, you'll need to change your kitchen and prepare it for your new lifestyle. This means giving away previous unhealthy foods and fats that are in your cupboard and updating your pantry and fridge to match your new eating habits. You might also need a few new pieces of equipment to help keep you on track. Some simple changes you can make are:

◆ Using lean cuts of meat
◆ Toss out and avoid buying processed foods
◆ Fill your fridge with fresh fruits and vegetables (recipes to follow)
◆ Experiment with soy milk, meat substitutes, and low-fat food items
◆ Switch to whole-grain and whole wheat
◆ Avoid frying when you're in the kitchen

There are also certain appliances that you can add to your kitchen to make cooking easier. It also helps facilitate your ability to make certain recipes. I highly suggest getting:

◆ **Microwave**—it can shorten the time it takes you to heat up leftovers and is an easy way to cook many vegetables as well.

◆ **A slow cooker.** When you can toss in some tasty vegetables and spices into a slow cooker and let them melt together until dinner time, it makes cooking very easy and very hands-off.

◆ **Freezer bags.** It's nice to make some things in bulk and freeze them for a later date. When you're in control of what you eat, you become more confident in eating your own leftovers.

◆ **Vegetable peeler.** Inevitably you are going to start eating more vegetables (I promise you'll find recipes that make them taste delicious in this cookbook). A peeler will make handling vegetables quick and easy.

◆ **A steamer.** Steaming vegetables is easy and it keeps them packed full of all their nutrients. I couldn't live without my steamer.

You might have to rearrange your kitchen, your diet, and your meal schedule. Yes, growing pains are inevitable. But there is a pot of gold at the end of this rainbow.

I found that I loved the changes I was making. It was easier to get up in the mornings, my body felt better, and I now have so much more energy to devote to my day. My biggest plus is that I didn't have to compromise on the taste or quality of my food. I still have a treat now and then that's not within the diabetic range, but learning portion control has helped me savor that treat rather than miss eating it as I once did.

I'm sure you'll find that within a month or two, you're loving these changes too.

Special Occasions and Other Challenges

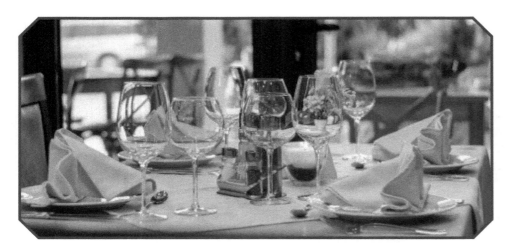

I know eating out can seem daunting. However, you don't need to be scared of it. Going to restaurants with friends, being on holiday, or attending conferences and events can put a kink in your dietary plan—but it doesn't have to.

1 Always plan ahead. If you're going to a restaurant see if you can find their menu online. Or call them to find out what kind of substitutions they allow or if they have boiled, steamed, or grilled options. If it's an event, try to find out as much as you can about the food being served.

2 Remember your portion sizes. If a restaurant doesn't offer a half portion, only eat half and take the rest of your meal home, or you could share your plate with a friend or partner. This keeps you from overeating when going out.

3 Don't be afraid to ask about substitutions. If they have a side salad instead of fries, switch it out. Ask them for their fat-free and low-sugar options for dressings and low-fat options for sauces. Most places cater to different diets nowadays.

4 Don't forget about what you're drinking. Try to avoid sugary drinks or overly sweetened drinks.

5 If you're with your friends and indulging in a glass of wine or beer is a must, then try to stick to light beers or dry wines. Those are best for diabetics.

6 You don't have to avoid dessert. Simply share it with a friend, or make sure that you save the room for the dessert calories in your diet. Eat a little less of your meal to incorporate the fats and calories from the dessert.

7 My ultimate tip is to move around. Park farthest away if you can and walk into the restaurant. It gives you some exercise and makes you feel like you earned that dessert afterward too!

Chapter 4: 21-Day Meal Plan

	BREAKFAST	LUNCH	DINNER	SNACK/DESSERTS
1	Carrot and Oat Pancakes [16]	Broiled Teriyaki Salmon [40]	Citrus Pork Tenderloin [60]	Apple Cinnamon Chimichanga [63]
2	Bacon-Wrapped Shrimps [21]	Chipotle Chili Pork [53]	Marinated Grilled Salmon with Lemongrass [39]	Chia and Raspberry Pudding [63]
3	Savory Breakfast Egg Bites [16]	Pork Diane [53]	Tartar Tuna Patties [41]	Sautéed Collard Greens and Cabbage [24]
4	Easy Caprese Skewers [22]	Blackened Spatchcock with Lime Aioli [49]	Lemon Parsley White Fish Fillets [41]	Crispy Apple Chips [62]
5	Simple Grain-Free Biscuits [15]	Fresh Rosemary Trout [42]	Citrus Chicken Thighs [46]	Roasted Delicata Squash with Thyme [24]
6	Cheesy Broccoli Bites [21]	Creamy and Aromatic Chicken [46]	Butter-Lemon Grilled Cod on Asparagus [42]	Date and Almond Balls with Seeds [62]
7	Brussels Sprout with Fried Eggs [15]	Cioppino (Seafood and Tomato Stew) [43]	Creamy and Cheesy Chicken Chile Casserole [47]	Roasted Asparagus and Red Peppers [25]
8	Simple Deviled Eggs [23]	Pork Souvlakia with Tzatziki Sauce [54]	Black Bean and Tomato Soup with Lime Yogurt [36]	Easy Banana Mug Cake [64]
9	Vanilla Coconut Pancakes [17]	Classic Texas Caviar [36]	Butternut Noodles With Mushroom Sauce [31]	Tarragon Spring Peas [25]
10	Kale Chips [23]	Beef, Tomato, and Pepper Tortillas [54]	Sautéed Zucchini and Tomatoes [29]	Pumpkin and Raspberry Muffins [64]

11	Cheesy Spinach and Egg Casserole [17]	Crispy Cowboy Black Bean Fritters [34]	Cheesy Mushroom and Pesto Flatbreads [30]	Apple Cinnamon Chimichanga [63]
12	Carrot and Oat Pancakes [16]	Classic Stroganoff [55]	Dandelion and Beet Greens [35]	Garlicky Mushrooms [27]
13	Scrumptious Orange Muffins [18]	Slow Cooked Beef and Vegetables Roast [57]	Homemade Vegetable Chili [31]	Chia and Raspberry Pudding [63]
14	Savory Breakfast Egg Bites [16]	Wilted Dandelion Greens with Sweet Onion [32]	Roasted Brussels Sprouts with Wild Rice Bowl [30]	Sesame Bok Choy with Almonds [28]
15	Easy Turkey Breakfast Patties [18]	Cilantro Lime Shrimp [44]	Turkey Meatball and Vegetable Kabobs [50]	Crispy Apple Chips [62]
16	Simple Grain-Free Biscuits [15]	Collard Greens with Tomato [32]	Panko Coconut Shrimp [44]	Lime Asparagus with Cashews [28]
17	Quick Breakfast Yogurt Sundae [20]	Easy Lime Lamb Cutlets [55]	Shrimp Coleslaw [45]	Date and Almond Balls with Seeds [62]
18	Cheesy Spinach and Egg Casserole [17]	Cheesy Summer Squash and Quinoa Casserole [33]	Roasted Chicken with Root Vegetables [48]	Apple Cinnamon Chimichanga [63]
19	Peanut Butter and Berry Oatmeal [19]	Creamy Macaroni and Cheese [33]	Ritzy Jerked Chicken Breasts [49]	Easy Banana Mug Cake [64]
20	Scrumptious Orange Muffins [18]	Roasted Tomato and Bell Pepper Soup [29]	Chicken with Carrot, and Kale [51]	Chia and Raspberry Pudding [63]
21	Pecan-Oatmeal Pancakes [19]	Spaghetti Puttanesca [34]	Sumptuous Lamb and Pomegranate Salad [52]	Pumpkin and Raspberry Muffins [64]

Chapter 5 Breakfast

Simple Grain-Free Biscuits

Prep time: 10 minutes | Cook time: 15 minutes | Serves 4

2 tablespoons unsalted butter
¼ cup plain low-fat Greek yogurt
Pinch salt
1½ cups finely ground almond flour

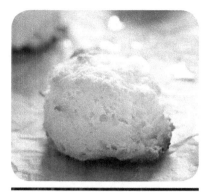

1. Preheat the oven to 375ºF (190ºC). Line a baking sheet with parchment paper and set aside.
2. Place the butter in a microwave-safe bowl and microwave for 15 to 20 seconds, or until it is just enough to soften.
3. Add the yogurt and salt to the bowl of butter and blend well.
4. Slowly pour in the almond flour and keep stirring until the mixture just comes together into a slightly sticky, shaggy dough.
5. Use a ¼-cup measuring cup to mound balls of dough onto the parchment-lined baking sheet and flatten each into a rounded biscuit shape, about 1 inch thick.
6. Bake in the preheated oven for 13 to 15 minutes, or until the biscuits are lightly golden brown.
7. Let the biscuits cool for 5 minutes before serving.

Tips: To add more flavors to these biscuits, you can serve them with a drizzle of honey or some fruit. They also taste great paired with a berry almond smoothie.

Per Serving
calories: 309 | fat: 28.1g
protein: 9.9g | carbs: 8.7g
fiber: 5.1g | sugar: 2.0g
sodium: 31mg

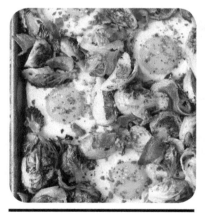

Tip: The Brussels sprouts, like other brassica vegetables, can be prepared ahead of time when you are free and kept in an airtight container in the refrigerator until ready to use.

Per Serving
calories: 157 | fat: 8.9g
protein: 10.1g | carbs: 11.8g
fiber: 4.1g | sugar: 4.0g
sodium: 233mg

Brussels Sprout with Fried Eggs

Prep time: 10 minutes | Cook time: 15 minutes | Serves 4

3 teaspoons extra-virgin olive oil, divided
1 pound (454 g) Brussels sprouts, sliced
2 garlic cloves, thinly sliced
¼ teaspoon salt
Juice of 1 lemon
4 eggs

1. Heat 1½ teaspoons of olive oil in a large skillet over medium heat.
2. Add the Brussels sprouts and sauté for 6 to 8 minutes until crispy and tender, stirring frequently.
3. Stir in the garlic and cook for about 1 minute until fragrant. Sprinkle with the salt and lemon juice.
4. Remove from the skillet to a plate and set aside.
5. Heat the remaining oil in the skillet over medium-high heat. Crack the eggs one at a time into the skillet and fry for about 3 minutes. Flip the eggs and continue cooking, or until the egg whites are set and the yolks are cooked to your liking.
6. Serve the fried eggs over the crispy Brussels sprouts.

Carrot and Oat Pancakes

Prep time: 10 minutes | Cook time: 8 minutes | Serves 4

¼ cup plain Greek yogurt
1 tablespoon pure maple syrup
1 cup rolled oats
1 cup low-fat cottage cheese
1 cup shredded carrots
½ cup unsweetened plain

almond milk
2 eggs
1 teaspoon baking powder
2 tablespoons ground flaxseed
½ teaspoon ground cinnamon
2 teaspoons canola oil, divided

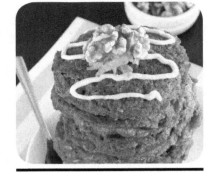

1. Stir together the yogurt and maple syrup in a small bowl and set aside.
2. Grind the oats in a blender, or until they are ground into a flour-like consistency.
3. Make the batter: Add the cheese, carrots, almond milk, eggs, baking powder, flaxseed, and cinnamon to the blender, and process until fully mixed and smooth.
4. Heat 1 teaspoon of canola oil in a large skillet over medium heat.
5. Make the pancakes: Pour ¼ cup of batter into the skillet and swirl the pan so the batter covers the bottom evenly. Cook for 1 to 2 minutes until bubbles form on the surface. Gently flip the pancake with a spatula and cook for 1 to 2 minutes more, or until the pancake turns golden brown around the edges. Repeat with the remaining canola oil and batter.
6. Top the pancakes with the maple yogurt and serve warm.

Tips: If you have a gluten sensitivity or allergy, you have to be very vigilant when selecting the oats. Make sure to select the oats that are labeled as "gluten free". You can decorate the pancakes with any topping of your choice, like heavy cream or blueberries.

Per Serving
calories: 227 | fat: 8.1g
protein: 14.9g | carbs: 24.2g
fiber: 4.0g | sugar: 7.0g
sodium: 403mg

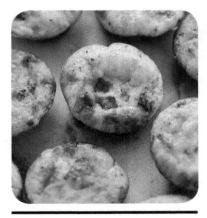

Tip: If you want to make a quick and easy breakfast, you can make these egg bites in single servings in the microwave.

Per Serving (1 Egg Bite)
calories: 68 | fat: 4.1g
protein: 6.2g | carbs: 2.9g
fiber: 1.1g | sugar: 2.0g
sodium: 126mg

Savory Breakfast Egg Bites

**Prep time: 10 minutes | Cook time: 20 to 25 minutes
Serves 8**

6 eggs, beaten
¼ cup unsweetened plain almond milk
¼ cup crumbled goat cheese
½ cup sliced brown mushrooms
1 cup chopped spinach

¼ cup sliced sun-dried tomatoes
1 red bell pepper, diced
Salt and freshly ground black pepper, to taste
Nonstick cooking spray

Special Equipment:
An 8-cup muffin tin

1. Preheat the oven to 350ºF (180ºC). Grease an 8-cup muffin tin with nonstick cooking spray.
2. Make the egg bites: Mix together the beaten eggs, almond milk, cheese, mushroom, spinach, tomatoes, bell pepper, salt, and pepper in a large bowl, and whisk to combine.
3. Spoon the mixture into the prepared muffin cups, filling each about three-quarters full.
4. Bake in the preheated oven for 20 to 25 minutes, or until the top is golden brown and a fork comes out clean.
5. Let the egg bites sit for 5 minutes until slightly cooled. Remove from the muffin tin and serve warm.

Vanilla Coconut Pancakes

Prep time: 5 minutes | Cook time: 15 minutes | Serves 4

½ cup coconut flour
1 teaspoon baking powder
½ teaspoon ground cinnamon
⅛ teaspoon salt
8 large eggs
⅓ cup unsweetened almond milk
2 tablespoons avocado or coconut oil
1 teaspoon vanilla extract

1. Stir together the flour, baking powder, cinnamon, and salt in a large bowl. Set aside.
2. Beat the eggs with the almond milk, oil, and vanilla in a medium bowl until fully mixed.
3. Heat a large nonstick skillet over medium-low heat.
4. Make the pancakes: Pour ⅓ cup of batter into the hot skillet, tilting the pan to spread it evenly. Cook for 3 to 4 minutes until bubbles form on the surface. Flip the pancake with a spatula and cook for about 3 minutes, or until the pancake is browned around the edges and cooked through. Repeat with the remaining batter.
5. Serve the pancakes on a plate while warm.

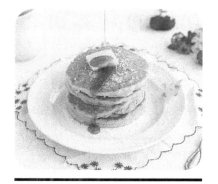

Tips: The water can be substituted for almond milk in this recipe, and you can use the butter instead of oil for a deeper flavor.

Per Serving
calories: 269 | fat: 17.8g
protein: 13.9g | carbs: 10.1g
fiber: 5.1g | sugar: 1.9g
sodium: 324mg

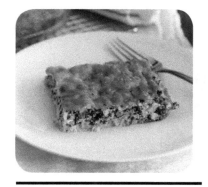

Tips: For a kick of spice, add a scant teaspoon of red pepper flakes to this meal. To add more flavors to this meal, you can serve it with a cup of your favorite berries.

Per Serving
calories: 105 | fat: 4.8g
protein: 8.9g | carbs: 6.1g
fiber: 1.7g | sugar: 1.0g
sodium: 486mg

Cheesy Spinach and Egg Casserole

Prep time: 10 minutes | Cook time: 35 minutes | Serves 8

1 (10-ounce / 284-g) package frozen spinach, thawed and drained
1 (14-ounce / 397-g) can artichoke hearts, drained
¼ cup finely chopped red bell pepper
8 eggs, lightly beaten
¼ cup unsweetened plain almond milk
2 garlic cloves, minced
½ teaspoon salt
½ teaspoon freshly ground black pepper
½ cup crumbled goat cheese
Nonstick cooking spray

1. Preheat the oven to 375ºF (190ºC). Spray a baking dish with nonstick cooking spray and set aside.
2. Mix the spinach, artichoke hearts, bell peppers, beaten eggs, almond milk, garlic, salt, and pepper in a large bowl, and stir to incorporate.
3. Pour the mixture into the greased baking dish and scatter the goat cheese on top.
4. Bake in the preheated oven for 35 minutes, or until the top is lightly golden around the edges and eggs are set.
5. Remove from the oven and serve warm.

Scrumptious Orange Muffins

Prep time: 15 minutes | Cook time: 15 minutes | Serves 8

Dry Ingredients:
2½ cups finely ground almond flour
½ teaspoon baking powder
½ teaspoon ground cardamom
¾ teaspoon ground cinnamon
¼ teaspoon salt

Wet Ingredients:
2 large eggs
4 tablespoons avocado or coconut oil
1 tablespoon raw honey
¼ teaspoon vanilla extract
Grated zest and juice of 1 medium orange

Special Equipment:
An 8-cup muffin tin

1. Preheat the oven to 375ºF (190ºC) and line an 8-cup muffin tin with paper liners.
2. Stir together the almond flour, baking powder, cardamon, cinnamon, and salt in a large bowl. Set aside.
3. Whisk together the eggs, oil, honey, vanilla, zest and juice in a medium bowl. Pour the mixture into the bowl of dry ingredients and stir with a spatula just until incorporated.
4. Pour the batter into the prepared muffin cups, filling each about three-quarters full.
5. Bake in the preheated oven for 15 minutes, or until the tops are golden and a toothpick inserted in the center comes out clean.
6. Let the muffins cool for 10 minutes before serving.

Tips: The honey can be replaced with 100% pure maple syrup in this recipe. They can be served with any toppings of your choice, such as fried eggs, bacon slices or shredded cheese.

Per Serving
calories: 287 | fat: 23.5g
protein: 7.9g | carbs: 15.8g
fiber: 3.8g | sugar: 9.8g
sodium: 96mg

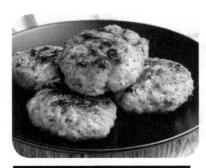

Easy Turkey Breakfast Patties

Prep time: 10 minutes | Cook time: 10 minutes | Serves 8

1 pound (454 g) lean ground turkey
½ teaspoon dried thyme
½ teaspoon dried sage
½ teaspoon salt
½ teaspoon freshly ground black pepper
¼ teaspoon ground fennel seeds
1 teaspoon extra-virgin olive oil

1. Mix the ground turkey, thyme, sage, salt, pepper, and fennel in a large bowl, and stir until well combined.
2. Form the turkey mixture into 8 equal-sized patties with your hands.
3. In a skillet, heat the olive oil over medium-high heat. Cook the patties for 3 to 4 minutes per side until cooked through.
4. Transfer the patties to a plate and serve hot.

Tip: The turkey patties perfectly go well with the pancakes for a wonderful weekend brunch.

Per Serving (1 Patty)
calories: 91 | fat: 4.8g
protein: 11.2g | carbs: 0.1g fiber: 0.1g | sugar: 0| sodium: 155mg

Pecan-Oatmeal Pancakes

Prep time: 10 minutes | Cook time: 15 minutes | Serves 6

1 cup quick-cooking oats
1½ teaspoons baking powder
2 eggs
⅓ cup mashed banana (about ½ medium banana)

⅓ cup skim milk
½ teaspoon vanilla extract
2 tablespoons chopped pecans
1 tablespoon canola oil

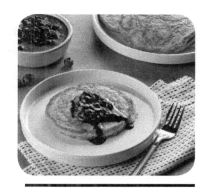

1. Pulse the oats in a food processor until they are ground into a powder-like consistency.
2. Transfer the ground oats to a small bowl, along with the baking powder. Mix well.
3. Whisk together the eggs, mashed banana, skim milk, and vanilla in another bowl. Pour into the bowl of dry ingredients and stir with a spatula just until well incorporated. Add the chopped pecans and mix well.
4. In a large nonstick skillet, heat the canola oil over medium heat.
5. Spoon ¼ cup of batter for each pancake onto the hot skillet, swirling the pan so the batter covers the bottom evenly. Cook for 1 to 2 minutes until bubbles form on top of the pancake. Flip the pancake and cook for an additional 1 to 2 minutes, or until the pancake is browned and cooked through. Repeat with the remaining batter.
6. Remove from the heat and serve on a plate.

Tip: To add more flavors to the pancake, you can add a pinch of salt to the batter and serve sprinkled with 1 teaspoon cinnamon, if desired.

Per Serving (1 Pancake)
calories: 131 | fat: 6.9g
protein: 5.2g | carbs: 13.1g
fiber: 2.0g | sugar: 2.9g
sodium: 120mg

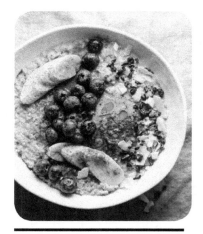

Tip: If you are sensitive to gluten, be sure to select the oats that are labeled as "gluten free".

Per Serving
calories: 260 | fat: 13.9g
protein: 10.1g | carbs: 26.9g
fiber: 7.1g | sugar: 1.0g
sodium: 130mg

Peanut Butter and Berry Oatmeal

Prep time: 5 minutes | Cook time: 15 minutes | Serves 2

1½ cups unsweetened vanilla almond milk
¾ cup rolled oats
1 tablespoon chia seeds
2 tablespoons natural peanut butter
¼ cup fresh berries, divided (optional)
2 tablespoons walnut pieces, divided (optional)

1. Add the almond milk, oats, and chia seeds to a small saucepan and bring to a boil.
2. Cover and continue cooking for about 10 minutes, stirring often, or until the oats have absorbed the milk.
3. Add the peanut butter and keep stirring until the oats are thick and creamy.
4. Divide the oatmeal into two serving bowls. Serve topped with the berries and walnut pieces, if desired.

Quick Breakfast Yogurt Sundae

Prep time: 5 minutes | Cook time: 0 minutes | Serves 1

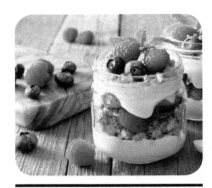

¾ cup plain Greek yogurt
¼ cup mixed berries (blueberries, strawberries, blackberries)
2 tablespoons cashew, walnut, or almond pieces
1 tablespoon ground flaxseed
2 fresh mint leaves, shredded

1. Pour the yogurt into a tall parfait glass and scatter the top with the berries, cashew pieces, and flaxseed.
2. Sprinkle the mint leaves on top for garnish and serve chilled.

Tips: The walnut or almond pieces can be substituted for the cashew. And if the fresh berries aren't available, the frozen will work too. Be sure to thaw and drain them properly.

Per Serving
calories: 238 | fat: 11.2g
protein: 20.9g | carbs: 15.8g
fiber: 4.1g | sugar: 8.9g
sodium: 63mg

Chapter 6 Appetizers

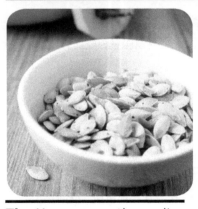

Aromatic Toasted Pumpkin Seeds

Prep time: 5 minutes | Cook time: 45 minutes | Serves 4

1 cup pumpkin seeds
1 teaspoon cinnamon
2 (0.04-ounce / 1-g) packets stevia
1 tablespoon canola oil
¼ teaspoon sea salt

1. Preheat the oven to 300°F (150°C).
2. Combine the pumpkin seeds with cinnamon, stevia, canola oil and salt in a bowl. Stir to mix well.
3. Pour the seeds in the single layer on a baking sheet, then arrange the sheet in the preheated oven.
4. Bake for 45 minutes or until well toasted and fragrant. Shake the sheet twice to bake the seeds evenly.
5. Serve immediately.

Tip: You can use the garlic powder, salt, and ground white pepper to replace the cinnamon and stevia for a distinct flavor of toasted pumpkin seeds.

Per Serving
calories: 202 | fat: 18.0g
protein: 8.8g | carbs: 5.1g
fiber: 2.3g | sugar: 0.4g
sodium: 151mg

Bacon-Wrapped Shrimps

Prep time: 10 minutes | Cook time: 6 minutes | Serves 10

20 shrimps, peeled and deveined
7 slices bacon, cut into 3 strips crosswise
4 leaves romaine lettuce

1. Preheat the oven to 400ºF (205ºC).
2. Wrap each shrimp with each bacon strip, then arrange the wrapped shrimps in a single layer on a baking sheet, seam side down.
3. Broil in the preheated oven for 6 minutes or until the bacon is well browned. Flip the shrimps halfway through the cooking time.
4. Remove the shrimps from the oven and serve on lettuce leaves.

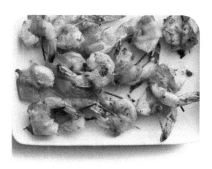

Tip: You can sprinkle the shrimps with garlic powder, cumin, ground oregano and black pepper when arranging in the baking sheet to herb the shrimps with more flavor.

Per Serving
calories: 70 | fat: 4.5g
protein: 7.0g | carbs:
0g fiber: 0g | sugar: 0g
sodium: 150mg

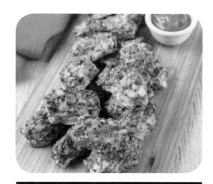

Tip: You can replace the broccoli with spinach, cauliflower, or kale for different cheesy bites.

Per Serving
calories: 100 | fat: 3.0g
protein: 7.0g | carbs: 13.0g
fiber: 3.0g | sugar: 3.0g
sodium: 250mg

Cheesy Broccoli Bites

Prep time: 10 minutes | Cook time: 25 minutes | Serves 6

2 tablespoons olive oil
2 heads broccoli, trimmed
1 eggs
$^1/_3$ cup reduced-fat shredded
Cheddar cheese
1 egg white
½ cup onion, chopped
$^1/_3$ cup bread crumbs
¼ teaspoon salt
¼ teaspoon black pepper

1. Preheat the oven to 400ºF (205ºC). Coat a large baking sheet with olive oil.
2. Arrange a colander in a saucepan, then place the broccoli in the colander. Pour the water in the saucepan to cover the bottom. Bring to a boil, then reduce the heat to low. Cover and simmer for 6 minutes or until the broccoli is fork-tender. Allow to cool for 10 minutes.
3. Put the broccoli and remaining ingredients in a food processor. Process to combine until lightly chunky. Let sit for 10 minutes.
4. Make the bites: Drop 1 tablespoon of the mixture on the baking sheet. Repeat with the remaining mixture.
5. Bake in the preheated oven for 25 minutes or until lightly browned. Flip the bites halfway through the cooking time.
6. Serve immediately.

Easy Caprese Skewers

Prep time: 5 minutes | Cook time: 0 minutes | Serves 2

12 cherry tomatoes
8 (1-inch) pieces Mozzarella cheese
12 basil leaves
¼ cup Italian Vinaigrette, for serving

Special Equipment:
4 wooden skewers, soaked in water for at least 30 minutes

1. Thread the tomatoes, cheese, and bay leaves alternatively through the skewers.
2. Place the skewers on a large plate and baste with the Italian Vinaigrette. Serve immediately.

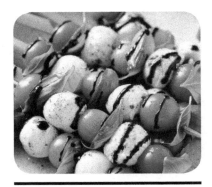

Tip: You can run the olives or cherry tomato on the skewers for more flavor.

Per Serving
calories: 230 | fat: 12.6g
protein: 21.3g | carbs: 8.5g
fiber: 1.9g | sugar: 4.9g
sodium: 672mg

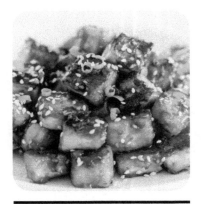

Tip: You can replace the applesauce with no-sugar-added apple-apricot sauce.

Per Serving
calories: 90 | fat: 6.0g
protein: 7.0g | carbs: 3.0g
fiber: 1.0g | sugar: 1.0g
sodium: 310mg

Grilled Tofu with Sesame Seeds

Prep time: 45 minutes | Cook time: 20 minutes | Serves 6

1½ tablespoons brown rice vinegar
1 scallion, green and white parts, minced
1 tablespoon ginger root, freshly grated
1 tablespoon no-sugar-added applesauce
2 tablespoons naturally brewed soy sauce
¼ teaspoon dried red pepper flakes, crushed
2 teaspoons sesame oil, toasted
1 (14-ounce / 397-g) package extra-firm tofu, drained and squeezed of excess liquid, cut into 18 pieces
2 tablespoons fresh cilantro
1 teaspoon toasted black or white sesame seeds

1. Combine the vinegar, scallion, ginger, applesauce, soy sauce, red pepper flakes, and sesame oil in a large bowl. Stir to mix well.
2. Dunk the tofu pieces in the bowl, then refrigerate to marinate for 30 minutes.
3. Preheat a grill pan over medium-high heat.
4. Place the tofu on the grill pan with tongs and reserve the marinade, then grill for 8 minutes or until the tofu is golden brown and has deep grilled marks on both sides. Flip the tofu halfway through the cooking time. You may need to work in batches to avoid overcrowding.
5. Transfer the tofu on a large plate and sprinkle with cilantro leaves and sesame seeds. Serve with the marinade alongside.

Kale Chips

Prep time: 5 minutes | Cook time: 15 minutes | Serves 1

¼ teaspoon garlic powder
Pinch cayenne, to taste
1 tablespoon extra-virgin olive oil
½ teaspoon sea salt, or to taste
1 (8-ounce / 227-g) bunch kale, trimmed and cut into 2-inch pieces, rinsed

1. Preheat the oven to 350ºF (180ºC). Line two baking sheets with parchment paper.
2. Combine the garlic powder, cayenne pepper, olive oil, and salt in a large bowl, then dunk the kale in the bowl. Toss to coat well.
3. Place the kale in the single layer on one of the baking sheet.
4. Arrange the sheet in the preheated oven and bake for 7 minutes. Remove the sheet from the oven and pour the kale in the single layer of the other baking sheet.
5. Move the sheet of kale back to the oven and bake for another 7 minutes or until the kale is crispy.
6. Serve immediately.

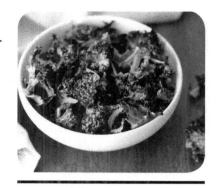

Tip: Sprinkle the kale with ground ginger and sesame seeds for a distinct flavor when tossing.

Per Serving
calories: 136 | fat: 14.0g
protein: 1.0g | carbs: 3.0g
fiber: 1.1g | sugar: 0.6g
sodium: 1170mg

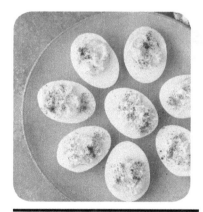

Tip: You can garnish the deviled eggs with cherry tomato slices, radish slices, or sprinkle with chopped scallions.

Per Serving
calories: 45 | fat: 3.0g
protein: 3.0g | carbs: 1.0g
fiber: 0g | sugar: 0g
sodium: 70mg

Simple Deviled Eggs

Prep time: 5 minutes | Cook time: 8 minutes | Serves 12

6 large eggs
⅛ teaspoon mustard powder
2 tablespoons plus 1 teaspoon light mayonnaise
Salt and freshly ground black pepper, to taste

1. Sit the eggs in a saucepan, then pour in enough water to cover the egg. Bring to a boil, then boil the eggs for another 8 minutes. Turn off the heat and cover, then let sit for 15 minutes.
2. Transfer the boiled eggs in a pot of cold water and peel under the water.
3. Transfer the eggs on a large plate, then cut in half. Remove the egg yolks and place them in a bowl, then mash with a fork.
4. Add the mustard powder, mayo, salt, and pepper to the bowl of yolks, then stir to mix well.
5. Spoon the yolk mixture in the egg white on the plate. Serve immediately.

Sautéed Collard Greens and Cabbage

Prep time: 10 minutes | Cook time: 10 minutes | Serves 8

2 tablespoons extra-virgin olive oil
1 collard greens bunch, stemmed and thinly sliced
½ small green cabbage, thinly sliced
6 garlic cloves, minced
1 tablespoon low-sodium soy sauce

1. Heat the olive oil in a large skillet over medium-high heat.
2. Sauté the collard greens in the oil for about 2 minutes, or until the greens start to wilt.
3. Toss in the cabbage and mix well. Reduce the heat to medium-low, cover, and cook for 5 to 7 minutes, stirring occasionally, or until the greens are softened.
4. Fold in the garlic and soy sauce and stir to combine. Cook for about 30 seconds more until fragrant.
5. Remove from the heat to a plate and serve.

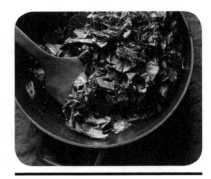

Tips: The low-sodium soy sauce can be replaced with tamari. To add more flavors to this dish, you can serve it with crisp bacon or potato salad.

Per Serving
calories: 73 | fat: 4.1g
protein: 3.2g | carbs: 5.9g
fiber: 2.9g | sugar: 0g
sodium: 128mg

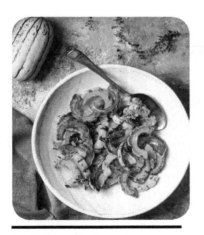

Tip: For a unique flavor, you can use your favorite spices such as cinnamon, oregano or rosemary instead of thyme.

Per Serving
calories: 78 | fat: 4.2g
protein: 1.1g | carbs: 11.8g
fiber: 2.1g | sugar: 2.9g
sodium: 122mg

Roasted Delicata Squash with Thyme

Prep time: 10 minutes | Cook time: 20 minutes | Serves 4

1 (1- to 1½-pound / 454- to 680-g) delicata squash, halved, seeded, and cut into ½-inch-thick strips
1 tablespoon extra-virgin olive oil
½ teaspoon dried thyme
¼ teaspoon salt
¼ teaspoon freshly ground black pepper

1. Preheat the oven to 400ºF (205ºC). Line a baking sheet with parchment paper and set aside.
2. Add the squash strips, olive oil, thyme, salt, and pepper in a large bowl, and toss until the squash strips are fully coated.
3. Place the squash strips on the prepared baking sheet in a single layer. Roast for about 20 minutes until lightly browned, flipping the strips halfway through.
4. Remove from the oven and serve on plates.

Roasted Asparagus and Red Peppers

Prep time: 5 minutes | Cook time: 15 minutes | Serves 4

1 pound (454 g) asparagus, woody ends trimmed, cut into 2-inch segments
2 red bell peppers, seeded, cut into 1-inch pieces
1 small onion, quartered
2 tablespoons Italian dressing

1. Preheat the oven to 400ºF (205ºC). Line a baking sheet with parchment paper and set aside.
2. Combine the asparagus with the peppers, onion, and dressing in a large bowl, and toss well.
3. Arrange the vegetables on the baking sheet and roast for about 15 minutes until softened. Flip the vegetables with a spatula once during cooking.
4. Transfer to a large platter and serve.

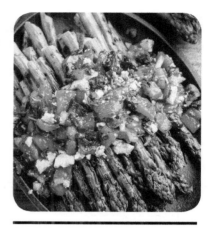

Tips: For even cooking, you can use the uniformly sized bunches of asparagus. To add more flavors to this dish, try adding slices of jalapeño peppers to Step 2.

Per Serving
calories: 92 | fat: 4.8g
protein: 2.9g | carbs: 10.7g
fiber: 4.0g | sugar: 5.7g
sodium: 31mg

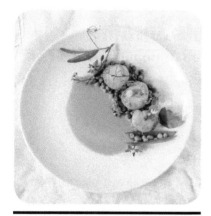

Tip: If you cannot find the fresh peas, the frozen peas work just as well.

Per Serving
calories: 82 | fat: 2.1g
protein: 4.2g | carbs: 12.0g
fiber: 3.8g | sugar: 4.9g
sodium: 48mg

Tarragon Spring Peas

Prep time: 10 minutes | Cook time: 12 minutes | Serves 6

1 tablespoon unsalted butter
½ Vidalia onion, thinly sliced
1 cup low-sodium vegetable broth
3 cups fresh shelled peas
1 tablespoon minced fresh tarragon

1. Melt the butter in a skillet over medium heat.
2. Sauté the onion in the melted butter for about 3 minutes until translucent, stirring occasionally.
3. Pour in the vegetable broth and whisk well. Add the peas and tarragon to the skillet and stir to combine.
4. Reduce the heat to low, cover, and cook for about 8 minutes more, or until the peas are tender.
5. Let the peas cool for 5 minutes and serve warm.

Butter-Orange Yams

Prep time: 7 minutes | Cook time: 45 minutes | Serves 8

2 medium jewel yams, cut into 2-inch dices
2 tablespoons unsalted butter
Juice of 1 large orange
1½ teaspoons ground cinnamon
¼ teaspoon ground ginger
¾ teaspoon ground nutmeg
⅛ teaspoon ground cloves

1. Preheat the oven to 350ºF (180ºC).
2. Arrange the yam dices on a rimmed baking sheet in a single layer. Set aside.
3. Add the butter, orange juice, cinnamon, ginger, nutmeg, and garlic cloves to a medium saucepan over medium-low heat. Cook for 3 to 5 minutes, stirring continuously, or until the sauce begins to thicken and bubble.
4. Spoon the sauce over the yams and toss to coat well.
5. Bake in the preheated oven for 40 minutes until tender.
6. Let the yams cool for 8 minutes on the baking sheet before removing and serving.

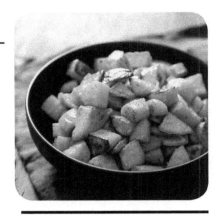

Tip: You can use ½ to ¾ cup bottled 100% orange juice to replace the fresh oranges in this recipe.

Per Serving
calories: 129 | fat: 2.8g
protein: 2.1g | carbs: 24.7g
fiber: 5.0g | sugar: 2.9g
sodium: 28mg

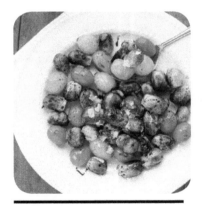

Tip: Be careful not to overcook the Brussels sprouts. If overcooked, their nutritional value will be reduced and Brussels sprouts will take on a bitter and sour taste.

Per Serving
calories: 111 | fat: 5.8g
protein: 5.0g | carbs: 13.7g
fiber: 4.9g | sugar: 2.7g
sodium: 103mg

Roasted Tomato Brussels Sprouts

Prep time: 15 minutes | Cook time: 20 minutes | Serves 4

1 pound (454 g) Brussels sprouts, trimmed and halved
1 tablespoon extra-virgin olive oil
Sea salt and freshly ground black pepper, to taste
½ cup sun-dried tomatoes, chopped
2 tablespoons freshly squeezed lemon juice
1 teaspoon lemon zest

1. Preheat the oven to 400ºF (205ºC). Line a large baking sheet with aluminum foil.
2. Toss the Brussels sprouts in the olive oil in a large bowl until well coated. Sprinkle with salt and pepper.
3. Spread out the seasoned Brussels sprouts on the prepared baking sheet in a single layer.
4. Roast in the preheated oven for 20 minutes, shaking the pan halfway through, or until the Brussels sprouts are crispy and browned on the outside.
5. Remove from the oven to a serving bowl. Add the tomatoes, lemon juice, and lemon zest, and stir to incorporate. Serve immediately.

Simple Sautéed Greens

Prep time: 10 minutes | Cook time: 10 minutes | Serves 4

2 tablespoons extra-virgin olive oil
1 pound (454 g) Swiss chard, coarse stems removed and leaves chopped
1 pound (454 g) kale, coarse stems removed and leaves chopped
½ teaspoon ground cardamom
1 tablespoon freshly squeezed lemon juice
Sea salt and freshly ground black pepper, to taste

1. Heat the olive oil in a large skillet over medium-high heat.
2. Add the Swiss chard, kale, cardamon, and lemon juice to the skillet, and stir to combine. Cook for about 10 minutes, stirring continuously, or until the greens are wilted.
3. Sprinkle with the salt and pepper and stir well.
4. Serve the greens on a plate while warm.

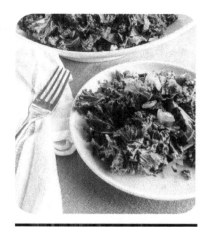

Tip: To add more flavors to this dish, you can serve it with your favorite pasta dish.

Per Serving
calories: 139 | fat: 6.8g
protein: 5.9g | carbs: 15.8g
fiber: 3.9g | sugar: 1.0g
sodium: 350mg

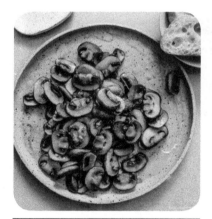

Tip: The mushrooms taste great paired with roasted pork tenderloin or grilled steaks.

Per Serving
calories: 96 | fat: 6.1g
protein: 6.9g | carbs: 8.2g
fiber: 1.7g | sugar: 3.9g
sodium: 91mg

Garlicky Mushrooms

Prep time: 10 minutes | Cook time: 12 minutes | Serves 4

1 tablespoon butter
2 teaspoons extra-virgin olive oil
2 pounds (907 g) button mushrooms, halved
2 teaspoons minced fresh garlic
1 teaspoon chopped fresh thyme
Sea salt and freshly ground black pepper, to taste

1. Heat the butter and olive oil in a large skillet over medium-high heat.
2. Add the mushrooms and sauté for 10 minutes, stirring occasionally, or until the mushrooms are lightly browned and cooked through.
3. Stir in the garlic and thyme and cook for an additional 2 minutes.
4. Season with salt and pepper and serve on a plate.

Sesame Bok Choy with Almonds

Prep time: 15 minutes | Cook time: 7 minutes | Serves 4

2 teaspoons sesame oil
2 pounds (907 g) bok choy, cleaned and quartered
2 teaspoons low-sodium soy sauce
Pinch red pepper flakes
½ cup toasted sliced almonds

1. Heat the sesame oil in a large skillet over medium heat until hot.
2. Sauté the bok choy in the hot oil for about 5 minutes, stirring occasionally, or until tender but still crisp.
3. Add the soy sauce and red pepper flakes and stir to combine. Continue sautéing for 2 minutes.
4. Transfer to a plate and serve topped with sliced almonds.

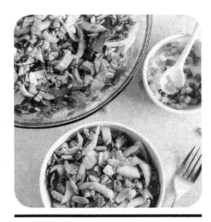

Tip: You can use the toasted sesame seeds to replace the almonds.

Per Serving
calories: 118 | fat: 7.8g
protein: 6.2g | carbs: 7.9g
fiber: 4.1g | sugar: 3.0g
sodium: 293mg

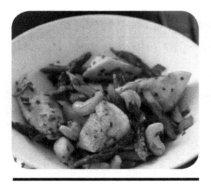

Tip: You can substitute the cashews with unsalted hazelnuts or pistachios.

Per Serving
calories: 173 | fat: 11.8g
protein: 8.0g | carbs: 43.7g
fiber: 4.9g | sugar: 5.0g
sodium: 65mg

Lime Asparagus with Cashews

**Prep time: 10 minutes | Cook time: 15 to 20 minutes
Serves 4**

2 pounds (907 g) asparagus, woody ends trimmed
1 tablespoon extra-virgin olive oil
Sea salt and freshly ground black pepper, to taste
½ cup chopped cashews
Zest and juice of 1 lime

1. Preheat the oven to 400ºF (205ºC). Line a baking sheet with aluminum foil.
2. Toss the asparagus with the olive oil in a medium bowl. Sprinkle the salt and pepper to season.
3. Arrange the asparagus on the baking sheet and bake for 15 to 20 minutes, or until lightly browned and tender.
4. Remove the asparagus from the oven to a serving bowl. Add the cashews, lime zest and juice, and toss to coat well. Serve immediately.

Chapter 8 Meatless Mains

Roasted Tomato and Bell Pepper Soup

Prep time: 20 minutes | Cook time: 35 minutes | Serves 6

2 tablespoons extra-virgin olive oil, plus more for coating the baking dish
16 plum tomatoes, cored and halved
4 celery stalks, coarsely chopped
4 red bell peppers, seeded, halved
4 garlic cloves, lightly crushed
1 sweet onion, cut into eighths
Sea salt and freshly ground black pepper, to taste
6 cups low-sodium chicken broth
2 tablespoons chopped fresh basil
2 ounces (57 g) goat cheese, grated

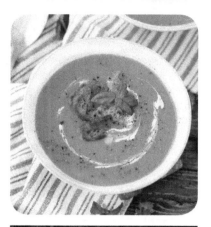

1. Preheat the oven to 400ºF (205ºC). Coat a large baking dish lightly with olive oil.
2. Put the tomatoes in the oiled dish, cut-side down. Scatter the celery, bell peppers, garlic, and onion on top of the tomatoes. Drizzle with 2 tablespoons of olive oil and season with salt and pepper.
3. Roast in the preheated oven for about 30 minutes, or until the vegetables are fork-tender and slightly charred.
4. Remove the vegetables from the oven. Let them rest for a few minutes until cooled slightly.
5. Transfer to a food processor, along with the chicken broth, and purée until fully mixed and smooth.
6. Pour the purée soup into a medium saucepan and bring it to a simmer over medium-high heat.
7. Sprinkle the basil and grated cheese on top before serving.

Tip: You can use the yellow and orange tomatoes to replace the plum tomatoes for a great source of lycopene.

Per Serving
calories: 187 | fat: 9.7g
protein: 7.8g | carbs: 21.3g
fiber: 6.1g | sugar: 14.0g
sodium: 825mg

Sautéed Zucchini and Tomatoes

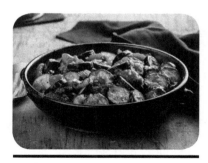

Tip: You can store the sautéed zucchini and tomatoes in the fridge for up to 4 days.

Per Serving
calories: 110 | fat: 4.4g
protein: 6.9g | carbs: 10.7g
fiber: 3.4g | sugar: 2.2g
sodium: 11mg

Prep time: 10 minutes | Cook time: 10 minutes | Serves 4

1 tablespoon vegetable oil
1 sliced onion
2 pounds (907 g) zucchini, peeled and cut into 1-inch-thick slices
2 tomatoes, chopped
1 green bell pepper, chopped
Salt and freshly ground black pepper, to taste

1. Heat the vegetable oil in a nonstick skillet until it shimmers.
2. Sauté the onion slices in the oil for about 3 minutes until translucent, stirring occasionally.
3. Add the zucchini, tomatoes, bell pepper, salt, and pepper to the skillet and stir to combine.
4. Reduce the heat, cover, and continue cooking for about 5 minutes, or until the veggies are tender.
5. Remove from the heat to a large plate and serve hot.

Roasted Brussels Sprouts with Wild Rice Bowl

Prep time: 15 minutes | Cook time: 12 minutes | Serves 4

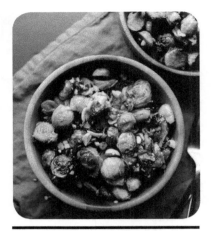

2 cups sliced Brussels sprouts
2 teaspoons plus 2 tablespoons extra-virgin olive oil
1 teaspoon Dijon mustard
Juice of 1 lemon
1 garlic clove, minced
½ teaspoon salt
¼ teaspoon freshly ground black pepper
1 cup sliced radishes
1 cup cooked wild rice
1 avocado, sliced

1. Preheat the oven to 400ºF (205ºC). Line a baking sheet with parchment paper and set aside.
2. Add 2 teaspoons of olive oil and Brussels sprouts to a medium bowl and toss to coat well.
3. Spread out the oiled Brussels sprouts on the prepared baking sheet. Roast in the preheated oven for 12 minutes, or until the Brussels sprouts are browned and crisp. Stir the Brussels sprouts once during cooking to ensure even cooking.
4. Meanwhile, make the dressing by whisking together the remaining olive oil, mustard, lemon juice, garlic, salt, and pepper in a small bowl.
5. Remove the Brussels sprouts from the oven to a large bowl. Add the radishes and cooked wild rice to the bowl. Drizzle with the prepared dressing and gently toss to coat everything evenly.
6. Divide the mixture into four bowls and scatter each bowl evenly with avocado slices. Serve immediately.

Tip: To add more flavors to this meal, try adding ½ cup shelled edamame or 4 ounces (113 g) of grilled tofu to the Brussels sprouts.

Per Serving
calories: 177 | fat: 10.7g
protein: 2.3g | carbs: 17.6g
fiber: 5.1g | sugar: 2.0g
sodium: 297mg

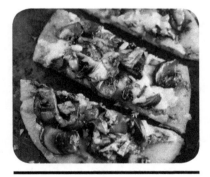

Cheesy Mushroom and Pesto Flatbreads

**Prep time: 5 minutes | Cook time: 13 to 17 minutes
Serves 2**

1 teaspoon extra-virgin olive oil
½ red onion, sliced
½ cup sliced mushrooms
Salt and freshly ground black pepper, to taste
¼ cup store-bought pesto sauce
2 whole-wheat flatbreads
¼ cup shredded Mozzarella cheese

1. Preheat the oven to 350ºF (180ºC).
2. Heat the olive oil in a small skillet over medium heat. Add the onion slices and mushrooms to the skillet, and sauté for 3 to 5 minutes, stirring occasionally, or until they start to soften. Season with salt and pepper.
3. Meanwhile, spoon 2 tablespoons of pesto sauce onto each flatbread and spread it all over. Evenly divide the mushroom mixture between two flatbreads, then scatter each top with 2 tablespoons of shredded cheese.
4. Transfer the flatbreads to a baking sheet and bake until the cheese melts and bubbles, about 10 to 12 minutes.
5. Let the flatbreads cool for 5 minutes and serve warm.

Tips: If the flatbread isn't available, the Ezekiel tortilla can be used as a substitute. For added flavor, you can serve with any of your favorite toppings, such as tomato slices, bell peppers or artichoke hearts.

Per Serving
calories: 346 | fat: 22.8g
protein: 14.2g | carbs: 27.6g
fiber: 7.3g | sugar: 4.0g
sodium: 790mg

Butternut Noodles With Mushroom Sauce

Prep time: 10 minutes | Cook time: 15 minutes | Serves 4

¼ cup extra-virgin olive oil
½ red onion, finely chopped
1 pound (454 g) cremini mushrooms, sliced
1 teaspoon dried thyme
½ teaspoon sea salt
3 garlic cloves, minced
½ cup dry white wine
Pinch red pepper flakes
4 cups butternut noodles
4 ounces (113 g) Parmesan cheese, grated (optional)

1. Heat the olive oil in a large skillet over medium-high heat until shimmering.
2. Add the onion, mushrooms, thyme, and salt to the skillet. Sauté for 6 minutes, stirring occasionally, or until the mushrooms begin to brown.
3. Stir in the garlic and cook for 30 seconds until fragrant.
4. Fold in the wine and red pepper flakes and whisk to combine.
5. Add the butternut noodles to the skillet and continue cooking for 5 minutes, stirring occasionally, or until the noodles are softened.
6. Divide the mixture among four bowls. Sprinkle the grated Parmesan cheese on top, if desired.

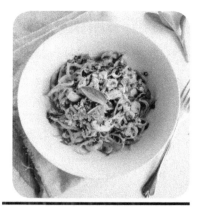

Tips: You can make the butternut noodles with a spiralizer, vegetable peeler or a knife. The zucchini noodles or shirataki noodles can be substituted for the butternut squash.

Per Serving
calories: 243 | fat: 14.2g
protein: 3.7g | carbs: 21.9g
fiber: 4.1g | sugar: 2.1g
sodium: 157mg

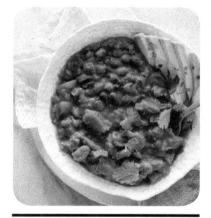

Tips: You can make a chili soup by adding 4 cups of vegetable broth. If you want to reduce the carbs, you can use half of the kidney beans in this recipe.

Per Serving
calories: 282 | fat: 10.1g
protein: 16.7g | carbs: 38.2g
fiber: 12.9g | sugar: 7.2g
sodium: 1128mg

Homemade Vegetable Chili

Prep time: 10 minutes | Cook time: 15 minutes | Serves 4

2 tablespoons extra-virgin olive oil
1 onion, finely chopped
1 green bell pepper, deseeded and chopped
1 (14-ounce / 397-g) can kidney beans, drained and rinsed
2 (14-ounce / 397-g) cans crushed tomatoes
2 cups veggie crumbles
1 teaspoon garlic powder
1 tablespoon chili powder
½ teaspoon sea salt

1. Heat the olive oil in a large skillet over medium-high heat until shimmering.
2. Add the onion and bell pepper and sauté for 5 minutes, stirring occasionally.
3. Fold in the beans, tomatoes, veggie crumbles, garlic powder, chili powder, and salt. Stir to incorporate and bring them to a simmer.
4. Reduce the heat and cook for an additional 5 minutes, stirring occasionally, or until the mixture is heated through.
5. Allow the mixture to cool for 5 minutes and serve warm.

Wilted Dandelion Greens with Sweet Onion

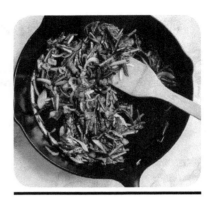

Prep time: 15 minutes | Cook time: 12 minutes | Serves 4

1 tablespoon extra-virgin olive oil
1 Vidalia onion, thinly sliced
2 garlic cloves, minced
2 bunches dandelion greens, roughly chopped
½ cup low-sodium vegetable broth
Freshly ground black pepper, to taste

1. Heat the olive oil in a large skillet over low heat.
2. Cook the onion and garlic for 2 to 3 minutes until tender, stirring occasionally.
3. Add the dandelion greens and broth and cook for 5 to 7 minutes, stirring frequently, or until the greens are wilted.
4. Transfer to a plate and season with black pepper. Serve warm.

Tips: Be sure to add more vegetable broth for preventing the onion and garlic from burning during cooking. For extra flavor and nutrition, you can add the dandelion greens to a white bean salad.

Per Serving
calories: 81 | fat: 3.8g
protein: 3.1g | carbs: 10.7g
fiber: 3.8g | sugar: 2.0g
sodium: 72mg

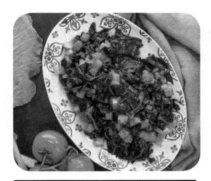

Tip: To add more flavors to this dish, serve it with pasta or cooked black beans and rice.

Per Serving
calories: 68 | fat: 2.1g
protein: 4.8g | carbs: 13.8g
fiber: 7.1g | sugar: 2.0g
sodium: 67mg

Collard Greens with Tomato

Prep time: 10 minutes | Cook time: 20 minutes | Serves 4

1 cup low-sodium vegetable broth, divided
½ onion, thinly sliced
2 garlic cloves, thinly sliced
1 medium tomato, chopped
1 large bunch collard greens including stems, roughly chopped
1 teaspoon ground cumin
½ teaspoon freshly ground black pepper

1. Add ½ cup of vegetable broth to a Dutch oven over medium heat and bring to a simmer.
2. Stir in the onion and garlic and cook for about 4 minutes until tender.
3. Add the remaining broth, tomato, greens, cumin, and pepper, and gently stir to combine.
4. Reduce the heat to low and simmer uncovered for 15 minutes. Serve warm.

Cheesy Summer Squash and Quinoa Casserole

Prep time: 15 minutes | Cook time: 27 to 30 minutes
Serves 8

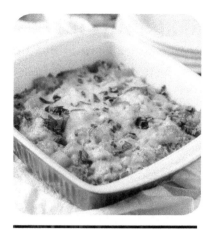

1 tablespoon extra-virgin olive oil
1 Vidalia onion, thinly sliced
1 large portobello mushroom, thinly sliced
6 yellow summer squash, thinly sliced
1 cup shredded Parmesan cheese, divided
1 cup shredded Cheddar cheese
½ cup tri-color quinoa
½ cup whole-wheat bread crumbs
1 tablespoon Creole seasoning

1. Preheat the oven to 350ºF (180ºC).
2. Heat the olive oil in a large cast iron pan over medium heat.
3. Sauté the onion, mushroom, and squash in the oil for 7 to 10 minutes, stirring occasionally, or until the vegetables are softened.
4. Remove from the heat and add ½ cup of Parmesan cheese and the Cheddar cheese to the vegetables. Stir well.
5. Mix together the quinoa, bread crumbs, the remaining Parmesan cheese, Creole seasoning in a small bowl, then scatter the mixture over the vegetables.
6. Place the cast iron pan in the preheated oven and bake until browned and cooked through, about 20 minutes.
7. Cool for 10 minutes and serve on plates while warm.

Tips: If you prefer a gluten-free dish, you can omit the bread crumbs in this recipe. It can be served as a wonderful lunch with a green salad or a tomato salad.

Per Serving
calories: 184 | fat: 8.9g
protein: 11.7g | carbs: 17.6g
fiber: 3.2g | sugar: 3.8g
sodium: 140mg

Creamy Macaroni and Cheese

Prep time: 10 minutes | Cook time: 25 minutes | Serves 6

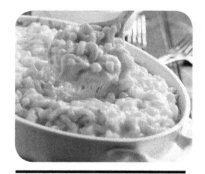

1 cup fat-free evaporated milk
½ cup skim milk
½ cup low-fat Cheddar cheese
½ cup low-fat cottage cheese
1 teaspoon nutmeg
Pinch cayenne pepper
Sea salt and freshly ground black pepper, to taste
6 cups cooked whole-wheat elbow macaroni
2 tablespoons grated Parmesan cheese

Tip: You can add other kinds of pasta instead of elbow macaroni to the cheese mixture.

Per Serving
calories: 245 | fat: 2.1g
protein: 15.7g | carbs: 43.8g
fiber: 3.8g | sugar: 6.8g
sodium: 186mg

1. Preheat the oven to 350ºF (180ºC).
2. Heat the milk in a large saucepan over low heat until it steams.
3. Add the Cheddar cheese and cottage cheese to the milk, and keep whisking, or until the cheese is melted.
4. Add the nutmeg and cayenne pepper and stir well. Sprinkle the salt and pepper to season.
5. Remove from the heat. Add the cooked macaroni to the cheese mixture and stir until well combined. Transfer the macaroni and cheese to a large casserole dish and top with the grated Parmesan cheese.
6. Bake in the preheated oven for about 20 minutes, or until bubbly and lightly browned.
7. Divide the macaroni and cheese among six bowls and serve.

Spaghetti Puttanesca

Prep time: 20 minutes | Cook time: 35 minutes | Serves 6

1 tablespoon extra-virgin olive oil
3 teaspoons minced garlic
1 sweet onion, chopped
2 celery stalks, chopped
2 (28-ounce / 794-g) cans sodium-free diced tomatoes
1 tablespoon chopped fresh oregano
2 tablespoons chopped fresh basil
½ teaspoon red pepper flakes
½ cup quartered, pitted Kalamata olives
¼ cup freshly squeezed lemon juice
8 ounces (227 g) cooked whole-wheat spaghetti

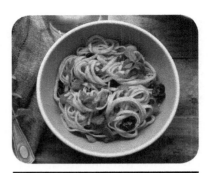

1. Heat the olive oil in a large saucepan over medium-high heat.
2. Add the garlic, onion, and celery to the saucepan and sauté for about 3 minutes, stirring occasionally, or until softened.
3. Toss in the tomatoes, oregano, basil, and pepper flakes and stir to combine. Allow the sauce to boil, stirring often to prevent from sticking to the bottom of the pan.
4. Reduce the heat to low and bring the sauce to a simmer, stirring occasionally, about 20 minutes.
5. Add the olives and lemon juice to the sauce and mix well.
6. Remove from the heat and spoon the sauce over the spaghetti. Toss well and serve warm.

Tip: You can add 2 tablespoons capers to the sauce and sprinkle with a small bunch of freshly chopped parsley before serving.

Per Serving
calories: 199 | fat: 4.7g
protein: 7.2g | carbs: 34.9g
fiber: 3.9g | sugar: 8.1g
sodium: 89mg

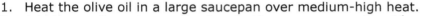

Chapter 9 Beans, Grains, and Legumes

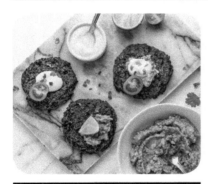

Crispy Cowboy Black Bean Fritters

Prep time: 10 minutes | Cook time: 25 minutes | Serves 20 Fritters

1¾ cups all-purpose flour
½ teaspoon cumin
2 teaspoons baking powder
2 teaspoons salt
½ teaspoon black pepper
4 egg whites, lightly beaten
1 cup salsa
2 (16-ounce / 454-g) cans no-salt-added black beans, rinsed and drained
1 tablespoon canola oil, plus extra if needed

Per Serving
calories: 115 | fat: 1.0g
protein: 6.0g | carbs: 20.0g
fiber: 5.0g | sugar: 2.0g
sodium: 350mg

1. Combine the flour, cumin, baking powder, salt, and pepper in a large bowl, then mix in the egg whites and salsa. Add the black beans and stir to mix well.
2. Heat the canola oil in a nonstick skillet over medium-high heat.
3. Spoon 1 teaspoon of the mixture into the skillet to make a fritter. Make more fritters to coat the bottom of the skillet. Keep a little space between each two fritters. You may need to work in batches to avoid overcrowding.
4. Cook for 3 minutes or until the fritters are golden brown on both sides. Flip the fritters and flatten with a spatula halfway through the cooking time. Repeat with the remaining mixture. Add more oil as needed.
5. Serve immediately.

Macaroni and Vegetable Pie

Prep time: 15 minutes | Cook time: 30 minutes | Serves 6

1 (1-pound / 454-g) package
whole-wheat macaroni
2 celery stalks, thinly sliced
1 small yellow onion, chopped
2 garlic cloves, minced
Salt, to taste
¼ teaspoon freshly ground
black pepper

2 tablespoons chickpea flour
2 cups grated reduced-fat
sharp Cheddar cheese
1 cup fat-free milk
2 large zucchini, finely grated
and squeezed dry
2 roasted red peppers,
chopped into ¼-inch pieces

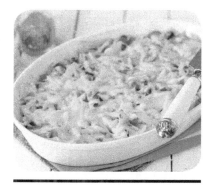

1. Preheat the oven to 350°F (180°C).
2. Bring a pot of water to a boil, then add the macaroni and cook for 4 minutes or until al dente.
3. Drain the macaroni and transfer to a large bowl. Reserve 1 cup of the macaroni water.
4. Pour the macaroni water in an oven-safe skillet and heat over medium heat.
5. Add the celery, onion, garlic, salt, and black pepper to the skillet and sauté for 4 minutes or until tender.
6. Gently mix in the chickpea flour, then fold in the cheese and milk. Keep stirring until the mixture is thick and smooth.
7. Add the cooked macaroni, zucchini, and red peppers. Stir to combine well.
8. Cover the skillet with aluminum foil and transfer it to the preheated oven.
9. Bake for 15 minutes or until the cheese melts, then remove the foil and bake for 5 more minutes or until lightly browned.
10. Remove the pie from the oven and serve immediately.

Tip: You can use the organic quinoa pasta to replace the macaroni to make this recipe gluten-free.

Per Serving
calories: 378 | fat: 4.0g
protein: 24.0g | carbs: 67.0g
fiber: 8.0g | sugar: 6.0g
sodium: 332mg

Dandelion and Beet Greens

Prep time: 10 minutes | Cook time: 15 minutes | Serves 4

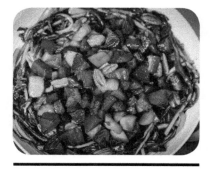

1 tablespoon olive oil
½ Vidalia onion, thinly sliced
1 bunch dandelion greens, cut into ribbons
1 bunch beet greens, cut into ribbons
½ cup low-sodium vegetable broth
1 (15-ounce / 425-g) can no-salt-added black beans
Salt and freshly ground black pepper, to taste

Tip: You can use collard greens, spinach, arugula, or Swiss chard to replace the beet greens or dandelion greens.

Per Serving
calories: 161 | fat: 4.0g
protein: 9.0g | carbs: 26.0g
fiber: 10.0g | sugar: 1.0g
sodium: 224mg

1. Heat the olive oil in a nonstick skillet over low heat until shimmering.
2. Add the onion and sauté for 3 minutes or until translucent.
3. Add the dandelion and beet greens, and broth to the skillet. Cover and cook for 8 minutes or until wilted.
4. Add the black beans and cook for 4 minutes or until soft. Sprinkle with salt and pepper. Stir to mix well.
5. Serve immediately.

Black Bean and Tomato Soup with Lime Yogurt

**Prep time: 8 hours 10 minutes | Cook time: 1 hour 33 minutes
Serves 8**

2 tablespoons avocado oil
1 medium onion, chopped
1 (10-ounce / 284-g) can diced tomatoes and green chilies
1 pound (454 g) dried black beans, soaked in water for at least 8 hours, rinsed
1 teaspoon ground cumin

3 garlic cloves, minced
6 cups chicken bone broth, vegetable broth, or water
Kosher salt, to taste
1 tablespoon freshly squeezed lime juice
¼ cup plain Greek yogurt

1. Heat the avocado oil in a nonstick skillet over medium heat until shimmering.
2. Add the onion and sauté for 3 minutes or until translucent.
3. Transfer the onion to a pot, then add the tomatoes and green chilies and their juices, black beans, cumin, garlic, broth, and salt. Stir to combine well.
4. Bring to a boil over medium-high heat, then reduce the heat to low. Simmer for 1 hour and 30 minutes or until the beans are soft.
5. Meanwhile, combine the lime juice with Greek yogurt in a small bowl. Stir to mix well.
6. Pour the soup in a large serving bowl, then drizzle with lime yogurt before serving.

Tip: If you want to make a thicker soup, remove 1 cup of beans from the pot after the simmering, then pour the remaining soup in a food processor. Process to purée the soup until smooth, then move 1 cup of beans back to the soup and serve.

Per Serving (1 Cup)
calories: 285 | fat: 6.0g
protein: 19.0g | carbs: 42.0g
fiber: 10.0g | sugar: 3.0g
sodium: 174mg

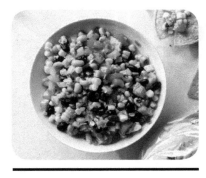

Classic Texas Caviar

Prep time: 10 minutes | Cook time: 0 minutes | Serves 6

For the Salad:
1 ear fresh corn, kernels removed
1 cup cooked lima beans
1 cup cooked black-eyed peas

1 red bell pepper, chopped
2 celery stalks, chopped
½ red onion, chopped

For the Dressing:
3 tablespoons apple cider vinegar
1 teaspoon paprika

2 tablespoons extra-virgin olive oil

Tip: You can replace the lima beans with the same amount of pinto beans for a distinct flavor.

Per Serving
calories: 170 | fat: 5.0g
protein: 10.0g | carbs: 29.0g
fiber: 10.0g | sugar: 4.0g
sodium: 20mg

Combine the corn, beans, peas, bell pepper, celery, and onion in a large bowl. Stir to mix well.
Combine the vinegar, paprika, and olive oil in a small bowl. Stir to combine well.
Pour the dressing into the salad and toss to mix well. Let sit for 20 minutes to infuse before serving.

Brown Rice with Carrot, and Scrambled Egg

Prep time: 15 minutes | Cook time: 20 minutes | Serves 4

1 tablespoon extra-virgin olive oil
1 bunch collard greens, stemmed and cut into chiffonade
1 carrot, cut into 2-inch matchsticks
1 red onion, thinly sliced
½ cup low-sodium vegetable broth
2 tablespoons coconut aminos
1 garlic clove, minced
1 cup cooked brown rice
1 large egg
1 teaspoon red pepper flakes
1 teaspoon paprika
Salt, to taste

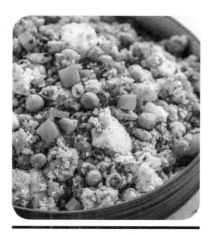

1. Heat the olive oil in a Dutch oven or a nonstick skillet over medium heat until shimmering.
2. Add the collard greens and sauté for 4 minutes or until wilted.
3. Add the carrot, onion, broth, coconut aminos, and garlic to the Dutch oven, then cover and cook 6 minutes or until the carrot is tender.
4. Add the brown rice and cook for 4 minutes. Keep stirring during the cooking.
5. Break the egg over them, then cook and scramble the egg for 4 minutes or until the egg is set.
6. Turn off the heat and sprinkle with red pepper flakes, paprika, and salt before serving.

Tip: You can use low-sodium soy sauce to replace the coconut aminos.

Per Serving
calories: 154 | fat: 6.0g
protein: 6.0g | carbs: 22.0g
fiber: 6.0g | sugar: 2.0g
sodium: 78mg

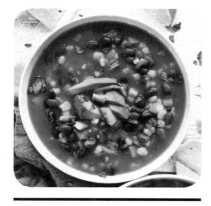

Black Bean, Corn, and Chicken Soup

Prep time: 10 minutes | Cook time: 25 minutes | Serves 7

2 tablespoons olive oil
½ onion, diced
1 pound (454 g) boneless and skinless chicken breast, cut into ½-inch cubes
½ teaspoon Adobo seasoning, divided
¼ teaspoon black pepper
1 (15-ounce / 425-g) can no-salt-added black beans, rinsed and drained
1 (14.5-ounce / 411-g) can fire-roasted tomatoes
½ cup frozen corn
½ teaspoon cumin
1 tablespoon chili powder
5 cups low-sodium chicken broth

Tip: You can use paprika, black pepper, onion powder, dried oregano, cumin, garlic powder, chili powder, and salt to make your own Adobo seasoning.

Per Serving
calories: 170 | fat: 3.5g
protein: 20.0g | carbs: 15.0g
fiber: 5.0g | sugar: 3.0g
sodium: 390mg

1. Grease a stockpot with olive oil and heat over medium-high heat until shimmering.
2. Add the onion and sauté for 3 minutes or until translucent.
3. Add the chicken breast and sprinkle with Adobo seasoning and pepper. Put the lid on and cook for 6 minutes or until lightly browned. Shake the pot halfway through the cooking time.
4. Add the remaining ingredients. Reduce the heat to low and simmer for 15 minutes or until the black beans are soft.
5. Serve immediately.

Wild Rice and Cranberries Salad

Prep time: 10 minutes | Cook time: 45 minutes
Serves 6 Cups

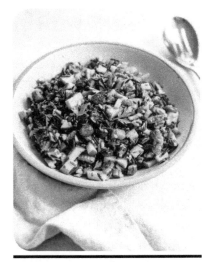

For the Rice:
2½ cups chicken bone broth, vegetable broth, or water

2 cups wild rice blend, rinsed
1 teaspoon kosher salt

For the Dressing:
Juice of 1 medium orange (about ¼ cup)
1½ teaspoons grated orange zest

¼ cup white wine vinegar
1 teaspoon pure maple syrup
¼ cup extra-virgin olive oil

For the Salad:
½ cup sliced almonds, toasted
¾ cup unsweetened dried cranberries

Freshly ground black pepper, to taste

Tip: You can combine the ingredients for the dressing in a jar and shake to combine. So you can keep the dressing and undressed salad in the refrigerate for future enjoyment.

Per Serving (¹/₃ Cup)
calories: 126 | fat: 5.0g
protein: 3.0g | carbs: 18.0g
fiber: 2.0g | sugar: 2.0g
sodium: 120mg

For the Rice
1. Pour the broth in a pot, then add the rice and sprinkle with salt. Bring to a boil over medium-high heat.
2. Reduce the heat to low. Cover the pot, then simmer for 45 minutes.
3. Turn off the heat and fluff the rice with a fork. Set aside until ready to use.

For the Dressing
1. When cooking the rice, make the dressing: Combine the ingredients for the dressing in a small bowl. Stir to combine well. Set aside until ready to use.

For the Salad
1. Put the cooked rice, almonds, and cranberries in a bowl, then sprinkle with black pepper. Add the dressing, then toss to combine well.
2. Serve immediately.

Red Kidney Beans with Tomatoes

Prep time: 10 minutes | Cook time: 8 to 12 minutes
Serves 8

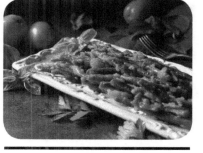

2 tablespoons olive oil
1 medium yellow onion, chopped
1 cup crushed tomatoes
2 garlic cloves, minced
2 cups low-sodium canned red kidney beans, rinsed
1 cup roughly chopped green beans
¼ cup low-sodium vegetable broth
1 teaspoon smoked paprika
Salt, to taste

1. Heat the olive oil in a nonstick skillet over medium heat until shimmering.
2. Add the onion, tomatoes, and garlic. Sauté for 3 to 5 minutes or until fragrant and the onion is translucent.
3. Add the kidney beans, green beans, and broth to the skillet. Sprinkle with paprika and salt, then sauté to combine well.
4. Cover the skillet and cook for 5 to 7 minutes or until the vegetables are tender. Serve immediately.

Tip: You can use the same amount of water to replace the vegetable broth.

Per Serving
calories: 187 | fat: 1.0g
protein: 13.0g | carbs: 34.0g
fiber: 10.0g | sugar: 4.0g
sodium: 102mg

Chapter 10 Fish and Seafood Mains

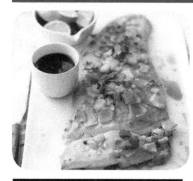

Marinated Grilled Salmon with Lemongrass

Prep time: 10 minutes | Cook time: 8 to 12 minutes
Serves 4

1 tablespoon olive oil
1 tablespoon grated fresh ginger
1 small hot chili pepper
1 tablespoon lemongrass, minced
2 tablespoons low-sodium soy sauce
1 tablespoon Splenda
4 (4-ounce / 113-g) skinless salmon fillets

1. Except for the salmon, stir together all the ingredients in a medium bowl. Brush the salmon fillets generously with the marinade and place in the fridge to marinate for 30 minutes.
2. Preheat the grill to medium heat.
3. Discard the marinade and transfer the salmon to the preheated grill.
4. Grill each side for 4 to 6 minutes, or until the fish is almost completely cooked through at the thickest part. Serve hot.

Tip: If you cannot find the lemongrass, you can substitute with 1 tablespoon lime juice.

Per Serving
calories: 223 | fat: 12.2g
protein: 25.7g | carbs: 2.0g
fiber: 0g | sugar: 2.9g
sodium: 203mg

Broiled Teriyaki Salmon

Prep time: 5 minutes | Cook time: 3 to 5 minutes
Serves 4

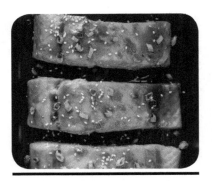

¹/₃ cup low-sodium soy sauce
¹/₃ cup pineapple juice
¼ cup water
2 tablespoons rice vinegar
1 garlic clove, minced
1 tablespoon honey

1 teaspoon peeled and grated fresh ginger
Pinch red pepper flakes
1 pound (454 g) salmon fillet, cut into 4 pieces

1. Preheat the oven broiler on high.
2. Stir together the soy sauce, pineapple juice, water, vinegar, garlic, honey, ginger, and red pepper flakes in a small bowl.
3. Marinate the fillets (flesh-side down) in the sauce for about 5 minutes.
4. Transfer the fillets (flesh-side up) to a rimmed baking sheet and brush them generously with any leftover sauce.
5. Broil the fish until it flakes apart easily and reaches an internal temperature of 145ºF (63ºC), about 3 to 5 minutes.
6. Let the fish cool for 5 minutes before serving.

Tips: If you want to make this dish gluten-free, you can use gluten-free soy sauce. And if the rice vinegar isn't available, just use the regular white vinegar.

Per Serving
calories: 201 | fat: 6.8g
protein: 23.7g | carbs: 8.9g
fiber: 1.0g | sugar: 10.2g
sodium: 750mg

Roasted Vegetable and Chicken Tortillas

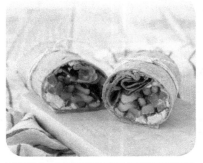

Prep time: 10 minutes | Cook time: 20 minutes | Serves 4

1 red bell pepper, seeded and cut into 1-inch-wide strips
½ small eggplant, cut into ¼-inch-thick slices
½ small red onion, sliced
1 medium zucchini, cut lengthwise into strips
1 tablespoon extra-virgin olive oil
Salt and freshly ground black pepper, to taste
4 whole-wheat tortilla wraps
2 (8-ounce / 227-g) cooked chicken breasts, sliced

Tip: How to cook the chicken breasts:
Preheat the oven to 400ºF (205ºC). Grease a baking sheet with 1 tablespoon olive oil. Place the chicken on the baking sheet and bake in the preheated oven for 24 minutes or until the internal temperature of the chicken reaches at least 165ºF (74ºC). Allow to cool before using.

1. Preheat the oven to 400ºF (205ºC). Line a baking sheet with aluminum foil.
2. Combine the bell pepper, eggplant, red onion, zucchini, and olive oil in a large bowl. Toss to coat well.
3. Pour the vegetables into the baking sheet, then sprinkle with salt and pepper.
4. Roast in the preheated oven for 20 minutes or until tender and charred.
5. Unfold the tortillas on a clean work surface, then divide the vegetables and chicken slices on the tortillas.
6. Wrap and serve immediately.

Per Serving
calories: 483 | fat: 25.0g
protein: 20.0g | carbs: 45.0g
fiber: 3.0g | sugar: 4.0g
sodium: 730mg

Tartar Tuna Patties

Prep time: 5 minutes | Cook time: 8 to 10 minutes
Serves 4

1 pound (454 g) canned tuna, drained
1 cup whole-wheat bread crumbs
2 large eggs, lightly beaten
Juice and zest of 1 lemon
½ onion, grated
1 tablespoon chopped fresh dill
3 tablespoons extra-virgin olive oil
½ cup tartar sauce, for topping

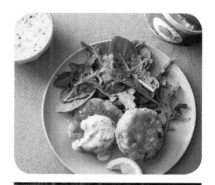

1. Mix together the tuna with the bread crumbs, beaten eggs, lemon juice and zest, onion, and dill in a large bowl, and stir until well incorporated.
2. Scoop out the tuna mixture and shape into 4 equal-sized patties with your hands.
3. Transfer the patties to a plate and chill in the refrigerator for 10 minutes.
4. Once chilled, heat the olive oil in a large nonstick skillet over medium-high heat.
5. Add the patties to the skillet and cook each side for 4 to 5 minutes, or until nicely browned on both sides.
6. Remove the patties from the heat and top with the tartar sauce.

Tips: For a distinct twist, try putting the patties on whole-grain toast slices as an open-faced sandwich. To make this a complete meal, serve the patties with a low-sugar vinaigrette.

Per Serving
calories: 529 | fat: 33.6g
protein: 34.9g | carbs: 18.3g
fiber: 2.1g | sugar: 3.8g
sodium: 673mg

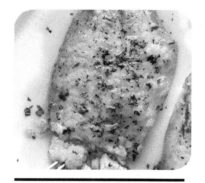

Tips: To make this a complete meal, you can serve it with roasted carrots and potatoes. It also goes well with the broccoli and spinach purée.

Per Serving
calories: 283 | fat: 17.2g
protein: 33.3g | carbs: 1.0g
fiber: 0g | sugar: 0g
sodium: 74mg

Lemon Parsley White Fish Fillets

Prep time: 10minutes | Cook time: 10 minutes | Serves 4

4 (6-ounce / 170-g) lean white fish fillets, rinsed and patted dry
Cooking spray
Paprika, to taste
Salt and pepper, to taste
2 tablespoons parsley, finely chopped
½ teaspoon lemon zest
¼ cup extra virgin olive oil
¼ teaspoon dried dill
1 medium lemon, halved

1. Preheat the oven to 400ºF (205ºC). Line a baking sheet with aluminum foil and spray with cooking spray.
2. Place the fillets on the foil and scatter with the paprika. Season as desired with salt and pepper.
3. Bake in the preheated oven for 10 minutes, or until the flesh flakes easily with a fork.
4. Meanwhile, stir together the parsley, lemon zest, olive oil, and dill in a small bowl.
5. Remove the fish from the oven to four plates. Squeeze the lemon juice over the fish and serve topped with the parsley mixture.

Fresh Rosemary Trout

Prep time: 5 minutes | Cook time: 7 to 8 minutes
Serves 2

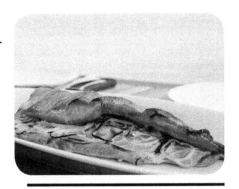

4 to 6 fresh rosemary sprigs
8 ounces (227 g) trout fillets, about ¼ inch thick; rinsed and patted dry
½ teaspoon olive oil
⅛ teaspoon salt
⅛ teaspoon pepper
1 teaspoon fresh lemon juice

1. Preheat the oven to 350ºF (180ºC).
2. Put the rosemary sprigs in a small baking pan in a single row. Spread the fillets on the top of the rosemary sprigs.
3. Brush both sides of each piece of fish with the olive oil. Sprinkle with the salt, pepper, and lemon juice.
4. Bake in the preheated oven for 7 to 8 minutes, or until the fish is opaque and flakes easily.
5. Divide the fillets between two plates and serve hot.

Tips: You can try this recipe with sole fillets in place of trout. The baked trout fillets taste great paired with zucchini noodles.

Per Serving
calories: 180 | fat: 9.1g
protein: 23.8g | carbs: 0g
fiber: 0g | sugar: 0g|
sodium: 210mg

Butter-Lemon Grilled Cod on Asparagus

Prep time: 5 minutes | Cook time: 9 to 12 minutes
Serves 4

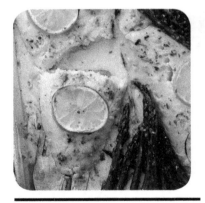

1 pound (454 g) asparagus spears, ends trimmed
Cooking spray
4 (4-ounce / 113-g) cod fillets, rinsed and patted dry
¼ teaspoon black pepper (optional)
¼ cup light butter with canola oil
Juice and zest of 1 medium lemon
¼ teaspoon salt (optional)

1. Heat a grill pan over medium-high heat.
2. Spray the asparagus spears with cooking spray. Cook the asparagus for 6 to 8 minutes until fork-tender, flipping occasionally.
3. Transfer to a large platter and keep warm.
4. Spray both sides of fillets with cooking spray. Season with ¼ teaspoon black pepper, if needed. Add the fillets to the pan and sear each side for 3 minutes until opaque.
5. Meantime, in a small bowl, whisk together the light butter, lemon zest, and ¼ teaspoon salt (if desired).
6. Spoon and spread the mixture all over the asparagus. Place the fish on top and squeeze the lemon juice over the fish. Serve immediately.

Tip: This dish can be eaten the way it is. However, you can serve the fish alongside other grilled or steamed vegetables.

Per Serving
calories: 158 | fat: 6.4g
protein: 23.0g | carbs: 6.1g
fiber: 3.0g | sugar: 2.8g
sodium: 212mg

Cioppino (Seafood and Tomato Stew)

Prep time: 10 minutes | Cook time: 15 minutes | Serves 4

2 tablespoons extra-virgin olive oil
1 onion, chopped finely
1 garlic clove, minced
½ cup dry white wine
1 (14-ounce / 397-g) can tomato sauce
8 ounces (227 g) shrimp, peeled and deveined
8 ounces (227 g) cod, pin bones removed and cut into 1-inch pieces
1 tablespoon Italian seasoning
½ teaspoon sea salt
Pinch red pepper flakes

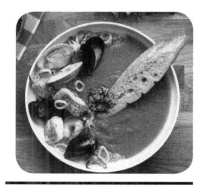

1. Heat the olive oil in a large skillet over medium-high heat until it shimmers.
2. Toss in the onion and cook for 3 minutes, stirring occasionally, or until the onion is translucent. Stir in the garlic and cook for 30 seconds until fragrant.
3. Add the wine and cook for 1 minute, stirring continuously.
4. Stir in the tomato sauce and bring the mixture to a simmer.
5. Add the shrimp and cod, Italian seasoning, salt, and red pepper flakes, and whisk to combine. Continue simmering for about 5 minutes, or until the fish is cooked through.
6. Remove from the heat and serve on plates.

Tips: If you prefer a heartier dish, try adding any of your favorite seafood, and you can add 1 cup of cooked white beans to your seafood.

Per Serving
calories: 242 | fat: 7.8g
protein: 23.2g | carbs: 10.7g
fiber: 2.1g | sugar: 7.7g
sodium:270mg

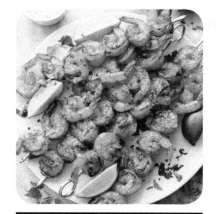

Tip: To add more favors to these shrimp skewers, you can serve with a drizzle of lime juice.

Per Serving
calories: 122 | fat: 0.8g
protein: 26.1g | carbs: 2.9g
fiber: 0.5g | sugar: 1.3g
sodium: 175mg

Grilled Shrimp Skewers with Yogurt

Prep time: 10 minutes | Cook time: 12 minutes | Serves 4

1 pound (454 g) shrimp, shelled and deveined
½ cup plain Greek yogurt
½ tablespoon chili paste
½ tablespoon lime juice
Chopped green onions, for garnish

Special Equipment:
Wooden skewers, soaked in water for at least 30 minutes

1. Thread the shrimp onto skewers, piercing once near the tail and once near the head. You can place about 5 shrimps on each skewer.
2. Preheat the grill to medium.
3. Place the shrimp skewers on the grill and cook for about 6 minutes, flipping the shrimp halfway through, or until the shrimp are totally pink and opaque.
4. Meanwhile, make the yogurt and chili sauce: In a small bowl, stir together the yogurt, chili paste, and lime juice.
5. Transfer the shrimp skewers to a large plate. Scatter the green onions on top for garnish and serve with the yogurt and chili sauce on the side.

Cilantro Lime Shrimp

Prep time: 15 minutes | Cook time: 8 minutes | Serves 4

1 teaspoon extra virgin olive oil
½ teaspoon garlic clove, minced
1 pound (454 g) large shrimp, peeled and deveined
¼ cup chopped fresh cilantro, or more to taste
1 lime, zested and juiced
¼ teaspoon salt
⅛ teaspoon black pepper

1. In a large heavy skillet, heat the olive oil over medium-high heat.
2. Add the minced garlic and cook for 30 seconds until fragrant.
3. Toss in the shrimp and cook for about 5 to 6 minutes, stirring occasionally, or until they turn pink and opaque.
4. Remove from the heat to a bowl. Add the cilantro, lime zest and juice, salt, and pepper to the shrimp, and toss to combine. Serve immediately.

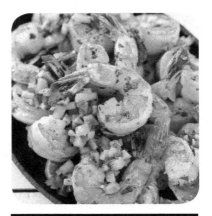

Tip: If you prefer a deep and rich flavor, you can double the garlic and serve sprinkled with lemon-pepper seasoning.

Per Serving
calories: 133 | fat: 3.5g
protein: 24.3g | carbs: 1.0g
fiber: 0g | sugar: 0g
sodium: 258mg

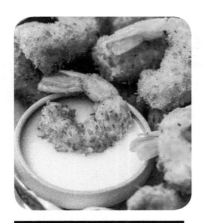

Tip: To add more flavors to this dish, serve the shrimp with sweet chili sauce and lime wedges.

Per Serving
calories: 181 | fat: 4.2g
protein: 27.8g | carbs: 9.0g
fiber: 2.3g | sugar: 0.8g
sodium: 227mg

Panko Coconut Shrimp

**Prep time: 12 minutes | Cook time: 6 to 8 minutes
Serves 4**

2 egg whites
1 tablespoon water
½ cup whole-wheat panko bread crumbs
¼ cup unsweetened coconut flakes
½ teaspoon turmeric
½ teaspoon ground coriander
½ teaspoon ground cumin
⅛ teaspoon salt
1 pound (454 g) large raw shrimp, peeled, deveined, and patted dry
Nonstick cooking spray

1. Preheat the air fry to 400ºF (205ºC).
2. In a shallow dish, beat the egg whites and water until slightly foamy. Set aside.
3. In a separate shallow dish, mix the bread crumbs, coconut flakes, turmeric, coriander, cumin, and salt, and stir until well combined.
4. Dredge the shrimp in the egg mixture, shaking off any excess, then coat them in the crumb-coconut mixture.
5. Spritz the air fryer basket with nonstick cooking spray and arrange the coated shrimp in the basket.
6. Air fry for 6 to 8 minutes, flipping the shrimp once during cooking, or until the shrimp are golden brown and cooked through.
7. Let the shrimp cool for 5 minutes before serving.

Shrimp Coleslaw

Prep time: 10 minutes | Cook time: 0 minutes | Serves 4

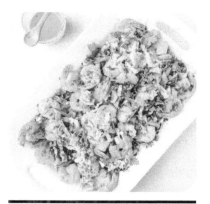

1 pound (454 g) frozen cooked shrimp, thawed
1 (8-ounce / 227-g) package shredded cabbage
3 tangerines, peeled and sectioned
3 scallions, sliced
3 tablespoons olive oil
2 teaspoons grated fresh ginger root
2 tablespoons white rice vinegar
⅛ teaspoon red pepper flakes
1 avocado, peeled, pitted, and sliced
¼ cup toasted slivered almonds (optional)
3 tablespoons chopped fresh cilantro

1. Stir together the shrimp, cabbage, tangerines, scallions, olive oil, ginger root, vinegar, and red pepper flakes in a large bowl.
2. Transfer to the refrigerator to chill for at least 30 minutes.
3. When ready to serve, sprinkle the avocado slices, almonds (if desired), and cilantro on top. Serve immediately.

Per Serving
calories: 362 | fat: 18.1g
protein: 29.6g | carbs: 20.5g
fiber: 5.4g | sugar: 8.3g
sodium: 138mg

Chapter 11 Poultry Mains

Herbed Chicken and Artichoke Hearts

Prep time: 10 minutes | Cook time: 20 minutes | Serves 4

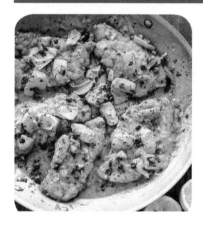

2 tablespoons olive oil, divided
4 (6-ounce / 170-g) boneless, skinless chicken breast halves
½ teaspoon dried thyme, divided
1 teaspoon crushed dried rosemary, divided
½ teaspoon ground black pepper, divided
2 (14-ounce / 397-g) cans water-packed, low-sodium
artichoke hearts, drained and quartered
½ cup low-sodium chicken broth
2 garlic cloves, chopped
1 medium onion, coarsely chopped
¼ cup shredded Parmesan cheese
1 lemon, cut into 8 slices
2 green onions, thinly sliced

Tip: You can replace the chicken broth with the same amount of white wine.

Per Serving
calories: 339 | fat: 9.0g
protein: 42.0g | carbs: 18.0g
fiber: 1.0g | sugar: 2.0g
sodium: 667mg

1. Preheat the oven to 375ºF (190ºC). Grease a baking sheet with 1 teaspoon of olive oil.
2. Place the chicken breasts on the baking sheet and rub with ¼ teaspoon of thyme, ½ teaspoon of rosemary, ¼ teaspoon of black pepper, and 1 tablespoon of olive oil.
3. Combine the artichoke hearts, chicken broth, garlic, onion, and remaining thyme, rosemary, black pepper, and olive oil. Toss to coat well.
4. Spread the artichoke around the chicken breasts, then scatter with Parmesan and lemon slices.
5. Place the baking sheet in the preheated oven and roast for 20 minutes or until the internal temperature of the chicken breasts reaches at least 165ºF (74ºC).
6. Remove the sheet from the oven. Allow to cool for 10 minutes, then serve with green onions on top.

Citrus Chicken Thighs

Prep time: 15 minutes | Cook time: 30 minutes | Serves 4

1 tablespoon grated fresh ginger
Sea salt, to taste
4 chicken thighs, bone-in, skinless
1 tablespoon extra-virgin olive oil
Juice and zest of ½ orange
Juice and zest of ½ lemon
1 tablespoon low-sodium soy sauce
Pinch red pepper flakes, to taste
2 tablespoons honey
1 tablespoon chopped fresh cilantro

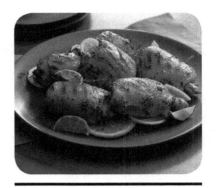

1. In a large bowl, combine the ginger and salt. Dunk the chicken thighs and toss to coat well.
2. Heat the olive oil in a nonstick skillet over medium-high heat until shimmering.
3. Add the chicken thighs and cook for 10 minutes or until well browned. Flip halfway through the cooking time.
4. Meanwhile, combine the orange juice and zest, lemon juice and zest, soy sauce, red pepper flakes, and honey. Stir to mix well.
5. Pour the mixture in the skillet. Reduce the heat to low, then cover and braise for 20 minutes. Add tablespoons of water if too dry.
6. Serve the chicken thighs garnished with cilantro.

Tip: To make this a complete meal, you can serve it with roasted asparagus and spinach and tomato soup.

Per Serving
calories: 114 | fat: 5.0g
protein: 9.0g | carbs: 9.0g
fiber: 0g | sugar: 9.0g
sodium: 287mg

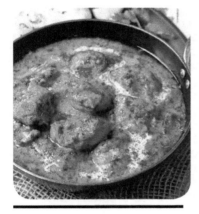

Tip: You can also garnish the chicken with black olives, sliced cherry tomatoes, or parsley for more flavor.

Per Serving
calories: 287 | fat: 14.0g
protein: 34.0g | carbs: 4.0g
fiber: 1.0g | sugar: 1.0g
sodium: 184mg

Creamy and Aromatic Chicken

Prep time: 15 minutes | Cook time: 30 minutes | Serves 4

4 (4-ounce / 113-g) boneless, skinless chicken breasts
Salt and freshly ground black pepper, to taste
1 tablespoon extra-virgin olive oil
½ sweet onion, chopped
2 teaspoons chopped fresh thyme
1 cup low-sodium chicken broth
¼ cup heavy whipping cream
1 scallion, white and green parts, chopped

1. Preheat the oven to 375ºF (190ºC).
2. On a clean work surface, rub the chicken with salt and pepper.
3. Heat the olive oil in an oven-safe skillet over medium-high heat until shimmering.
4. Put the chicken in the skillet and cook for 10 minutes or until well browned. Flip halfway through. Transfer onto a platter and set aside.
5. Add the onion to the skillet and sauté for 3 minutes or until translucent.
6. Add the thyme and broth and simmer for 6 minutes or until the liquid reduces in half.
7. Mix in the cream, then put the chicken back to the skillet.
8. Arrange the skillet in the oven and bake for 10 minutes.
9. Remove the skillet from the oven and serve them with scallion.

Creamy and Cheesy Chicken Chile Casserole

Prep time: 25 minutes | Cook time: 32 minutes | Serves 4

1 tablespoon olive oil
4 eggs, beaten
3 tablespoons softened cream cheese
¾ cup heavy whipping cream
1 teaspoon cumin
½ garlic powder
½ teaspoon salt
½ teaspoon ground black pepper
2 (6- to 8-ounce / 170- to

227-g) chicken breast, cooked and shredded
4 large whole green chiles, rinsed and patted dry, flattened
1 cup shredded Jack cheese
1 cup shredded Cheddar cheese
¼ teaspoon red pepper flakes, optional

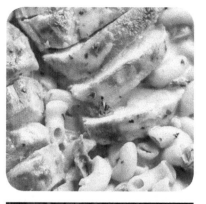

Tip: To make this a complete meal, you can serve it with arugula salad and gazpacho.

Per Serving
calories: 412 | fat: 30.0g
protein: 30.0g | carbs: 4.0g
fiber: 1.0g | sugar: 1.0g
sodium: 727mg

1. Preheat the oven to 350ºF (180ºC). Grease a casserole dish with olive oil.
2. Combine the eggs, cream cheese, cream, cumin, garlic powder, salt, and black pepper in a large bowl. Stir to mix well.
3. Dunk the chicken in the mixture. Press to coat well. Set aside.
4. Lay two chiles on the casserole dish, then flatten to cover the bottom. Pour half of the cream chicken mixture over the chiles.
5. Scatter ½ cup of Jack cheese and ½ cup of Cheddar cheese on the cream chicken, then top them with remaining two flattened chiles.
6. Pour the remaining cream chicken mixture over, then scatter the remaining cheeses and sprinkle them with red pepper flakes.
7. Arrange the casserole dish in the preheated oven and bake for 30 minutes, then turn the oven to broil for 2 minutes until the top of the casserole is well browned.
8. Remove the casserole from the oven. Allow to cool for 15 minutes, then serve warm.

Roasted Chicken with Root Vegetables

Prep time: 20 minutes | Cook time: 41 minutes | Serves 6

1 teaspoon minced fresh rosemary
1 teaspoon minced fresh thyme
1 teaspoon salt
1 teaspoon ground black pepper
2 tablespoons olive oil, divided
6 (6-ounce / 170-g) boneless, skinless chicken breast halves
2 medium fennel bulbs, chopped
4 medium peeled carrots, chopped
3 peeled medium radishes, chopped
3 tablespoons honey
½ cup white wine
2 cups chicken stock
3 bay leaves

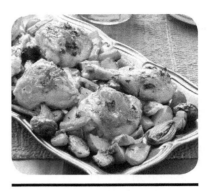

Tip: To make this a complete meal, you can serve it with creamy scallop soup.

Per Serving
calories: 364 | fat: 10.2g
protein: 41.8g | carbs: 22.2g
fiber: 3.8g | sugar: 15.1g
sodium: 650mg

1. Preheat the oven to 375ºF (190ºC).
2. Mix the rosemary, thyme, salt, and black pepper in a small bowl.
3. Heat 1 tablespoon of olive oil in a nonstick skillet over medium-high heat until shimmering.
4. On a clean work surface, rub the chicken breasts with half of the seasoning mixture.
5. Place the chicken in the skillet and cook for 6 minutes or until lightly browned on both sides. Remove the chicken from the skillet and set aside.
6. Mix the fennel bulbs, carrots, and radishes in a microwave-safe bowl, then sprinkle with remaining seasoning mixture and drizzle with honey, white wine, and remaining olive oil. Toss to combine well.
7. Cover the bowl and microwave the root vegetables for 10 minutes or until soft.
8. Arrange the root vegetables and chicken in a baking sheet, then pour in the chicken stock and honey mixture remains in the bowl. Top them with bay leaves.
9. Place the sheet in the preheated oven and roast for 25 minutes or until the internal temperature of the chicken reaches at least 165ºF (74ºC).
10. Remove the sheet from the oven and transfer the chicken and vegetables on a large plate. Discard the bay leaves, then allow to cool for a few minutes before serving.

Ritzy Jerked Chicken Breasts

Prep time: 4 hours 10 minutes | Cook time: 15 minutes
Serves 4

2 habanero chile peppers, halved lengthwise, seeded
½ sweet onion, cut into chunks
1 tablespoon minced garlic
1 tablespoon ground allspice
2 teaspoons chopped fresh thyme
¼ cup freshly squeezed lime juice
½ teaspoon ground nutmeg
¼ teaspoon ground cinnamon
1 teaspoon freshly ground black pepper
2 tablespoons extra-virgin olive oil
4 (5-ounce / 142-g) boneless, skinless chicken breasts
2 cups fresh arugula
1 cup halved cherry tomatoes

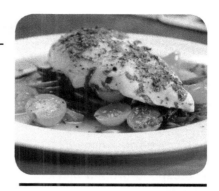

1. Combine the habaneros, onion, garlic, allspice, thyme, lime juice, nutmeg, cinnamon, black pepper, and olive oil in a blender. Pulse to blender well.
2. Transfer the mixture into a large bowl or two medium bowls, then dunk the chicken in the bowl and press to coat well.
3. Put the bowl in the refrigerator and marinate for at least 4 hours.
4. Preheat the oven to 400ºF (205ºC).
5. Remove the bowl from the refrigerator, then discard the marinade.
6. Arrange the chicken on a baking sheet, then roast in the preheated oven for 15 minutes or until golden brown and lightly charred. Flip the chicken halfway through the cooking time.
7. Remove the baking sheet from the oven and let sit for 5 minutes. Transfer the chicken on a large plate and serve with arugula and cherry tomatoes.

Tip: You can use the same amount of blanched spinach to replace the arugula to serve with the chicken.

Per Serving
calories: 226 | fat: 9.0g
protein: 33.0g | carbs: 3.0g
fiber: 0g | sugar: 1.0g
sodium: 92mg

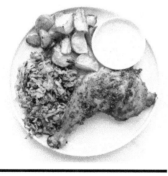

Tip: To make this a complete meal, you can serve it with roasted Brussels sprouts or radish soup.

Per Serving
calories: 436 | fat: 16.3g
protein: 61.8g | carbs: 6.8g
fiber: 0.7g | sugar: 1.5g
sodium: 653mg

Blackened Spatchcock with Lime Aioli

Prep time: 15 minutes | Cook time: 45 minutes | Serves 6

4 pounds (1.8 kg) chicken, spatchcocked
3 tablespoons blackened seasoning
2 tablespoons olive oil

Lime Aioli:
½ cup mayonnaise
Juice and zest of 1 lime
¼ teaspoon kosher salt
¼ teaspoon ground black pepper

1. Preheat the grill to medium high heat.
2. On a clean work surface, rub the chicken with blackened seasoning and olive oil.
3. Place the chicken on the preheated grill, skin side up, and grill for 45 minutes or until the internal temperature of the chicken reaches at least 165ºF (74ºC).
4. Meanwhile, combine the ingredients for the aioli in a small bowl and stir to mix well.
5. Once the chicken is fully grilled, transfer it to a large plate and baste with the lime aioli. Allow to cool and serve.

Turkey Meatball and Vegetable Kabobs

Prep time: 50 minutes | Cook time: 20 minutes | Serves 6

20 ounces (567 g) lean ground turkey (93% fat-free)
2 egg whites
2 tablespoons grated Parmesan cheese
2 cloves garlic, minced
½ teaspoon salt, or to taste
¼ teaspoon ground black pepper
1 tablespoon olive oil
8 ounces (227 g) fresh cremini mushrooms, cut in half to make 12 pieces
24 cherry tomatoes
1 medium onion, cut into 12 pieces
¼ cup balsamic vinegar

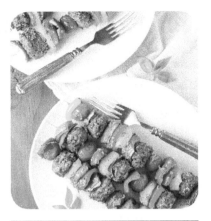

Special Equipment:
12 bamboo skewers, soaked in water for at least 30 minutes

1. Mix the ground turkey, egg whites, Parmesan, garlic, salt, and pepper in a large bowl. Stir to combine well.
2. Shape the mixture into 12 meatballs and place on a baking sheet. Refrigerate for at least 30 minutes.
3. Preheat the oven to 375ºF (190ºC). Grease another baking sheet with 1 tablespoon of olive oil.
4. Remove the meatballs from the refrigerator. Run the bamboo skewers through 2 meatballs, 1 mushroom, 2 cherry tomatoes, and 1 onion piece alternatively.
5. Arrange the kabobs on the greased baking sheet and brush with balsamic vinegar.
6. Grill in the preheated oven for 20 minutes or until an instant-read thermometer inserted in the middle of the meatballs reads at least 165ºF (74ºC). Flip the kabobs halfway through the cooking time.
7. Allow the kabobs to cool for 10 minutes, then serve warm.

Tips: You can use grape tomatoes to replace cherry tomatoes.
You can reserve half of the balsamic vinegar when brushing the kabobs, then brush the kabobs with reserved balsamic vinegar and more olive oil when flipping. This will help to grill the kabobs evenly.

Per Serving
calories: 200 | fat: 8.0g
protein: 22.0g | carbs: 7.0g
fiber: 1.0g | sugar: 4.0g
sodium: 120mg

Chicken with Carrot, and Kale

Prep time: 15 minutes | Cook time: 27 minutes | Serves 2

½ cup couscous
1 cup water, divided
⅓ cup basil pesto
3 teaspoons olive oil, divided
3 (2-ounce / 57-g) whole
carrots, rinsed, thinly sliced
Salt and ground black pepper,
to taste
1 (about 6-ounce / 170-g)

bunch kale, rinsed, stems
removed, chopped
2 cloves garlic, minced
2 tablespoons dried currants
1 tablespoon red wine vinegar
2 (6-ounce / 170-g) boneless,
skinless chicken breasts,
rinsed
1 tablespoon Italian seasoning

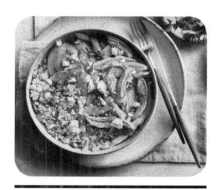

Tip: To make this a complete meal, you can serve it with beef stew or leafy green salad.

Per Serving
calories: 461 | fat: 14.2g
protein: 57.0g | carbs: 26.1g
fiber: 6.5g | sugar: 5.0g
sodium: 1210mg

1. Pour the couscous and ¾ cup of water in a pot. Bring to a boil on high heat. Reduce the heat to low. Simmer for 7 minutes or until most of the water has been absorbed. Fluffy with a fork and mix in the basil pesto.
2. Heat 1 teaspoon of olive oil in a nonstick skillet over medium-high heat until shimmering.
3. Add the carrots, then sprinkle with salt and pepper. Sauté for 3 minutes or until tender.
4. Add the kale and garlic and sauté for 2 minutes or until the kale is lightly wilted.
5. Add the currents and remaining water and sauté for 3 minutes or until most of the water is cooked off.
6. Turn off the heat, then mix in the red wine vinegar. Transfer them in a large bowl and cover to keep warm.
7. On a clean work surface, rub the chicken with Italian seasoning, salt, and pepper.
8. Clean the skillet and heat 2 teaspoons of olive oil over medium-high heat until shimmering.
9. Add the chicken and sear for 12 minutes or until well browned. Flip the chicken halfway through the cooking time.
10. Transfer the chicken to a large plate, then spread with vegetables and couscous. Slice to serve.

Sumptuous Lamb and Pomegranate Salad

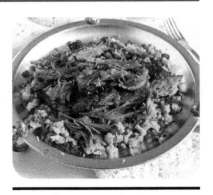

Prep time: 8 hours 35 minutes | Cook time: 30 minutes
Serves 8

1½ cups pomegranate juice
4 tablespoons olive oil, divided
1 tablespoon ground cinnamon
1 teaspoon cumin
1 tablespoon ground ginger
3 cloves garlic, chopped
Salt and freshly ground black pepper, to taste
1 (4-pound / 1.8-kg) lamb leg, deboned, butterflied, and fat trimmed
2 tablespoons pomegranate balsamic vinegar
2 teaspoons Dijon mustard
½ cup pomegranate seeds
5 cups baby kale
4 cups fresh green beans, blanched
¼ cup toasted walnut halves
2 fennel bulbs, thinly sliced
2 tablespoons Gorgonzola cheese

Tips: You can use the same amount of sliced red grapes to replace the pomegranate seeds. If you don't have pomegranate balsamic vinegar, you can juice use the balsamic vinegar to replace it.

Per Serving
calories: 380 | fat: 21.0g
protein: 32.0g | carbs: 16.0g
fiber: 5.0g | sugar: 6.0g
sodium: 240mg

1. Mix the pomegranate juice, 1 tablespoon of olive oil, cinnamon, cumin, ginger, garlic, salt, and black pepper in a large bowl. Stir to mix well.
2. Dunk the lamb leg in the mixture, press to coat well. Wrap the bowl in plastic and refrigerate to marinate for at least 8 hours.
3. Remove the bowl from the refrigerate and let sit for 20 minutes. Pat the lamb dry with paper towels.
4. Preheat the grill to high heat.
5. Brush the grill grates with 1 tablespoon of olive oil, then arrange the lamb on the grill grates.
6. Grill for 30 minutes or until the internal temperature of the lamb reaches at least 145ºF (63ºC). Flip the lamb halfway through the cooking time.
7. Remove the lamb from the grill and wrap with aluminum foil. Let stand for 15 minutes.
8. Meanwhile, Combine the vinegar, mustard, salt, black pepper, and remaining olive oil in a separate large bowl. Stir to mix well.
9. Add the remaining ingredients and lamb leg to the bowl and toss to combine well. Serve immediately.

Chipotle Chili Pork

Prep time: 4 hours 20 minutes | Cook time: 20 minutes
Serves 4

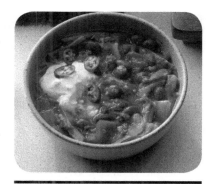

4 (5-ounce / 142-g) pork chops, about 1 inch thick
1 tablespoon chipotle chili powder
Juice and zest of 1 lime
2 teaspoons minced garlic
1 teaspoon ground cinnamon
1 tablespoon extra-virgin olive oil
Pinch sea salt
Lime wedges, for garnish

1. Combine all the ingredients, except for the lemon wedges, in a large bowl. Toss to combine well.
2. Wrap the bowl in plastic and refrigerate to marinate for at least 4 hours.
3. Preheat the oven to 400ºF (205ºC). Set a rack on a baking sheet.
4. Remove the bowl from the refrigerator and let sit for 15 minutes. Discard the marinade and place the pork on the rack.
5. Roast in the preheated oven for 20 minutes or until well browned. Flip the pork halfway through the cooking time.
6. Serve immediately with lime wedges.

Tip: You can use crushed chipotle pepper, paprika, cumin, garlic powder, and oregano to make your own chipotle chili powder.

Per Serving
calories: 204 | fat: 9.0g
protein: 30.0g | carbs: 1.0g
fiber: 0g | sugar: 1.0g
sodium: 317mg

Pork Diane

Prep time: 10 minutes | Cook time: 20 minutes | Serves 4

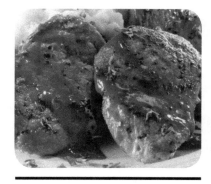

Tip: To make this recipe a complete meal, you can serve it with zucchini and cucumber salad or lettuce salad.

Per Serving
calories: 200 | fat: 8.0g
protein: 30.0g | carbs: 1.0g
fiber: 0g | sugar: 1.0g
sodium: 394mg

2 teaspoons Worcestershire sauce
1 tablespoon freshly squeezed lemon juice
¼ cup low-sodium chicken broth
2 teaspoons Dijon mustard
4 (5-ounce / 142-g) boneless pork top loin chops, about 1 inch thick
Sea salt and freshly ground black pepper, to taste
1 teaspoon extra-virgin olive oil
2 teaspoons chopped fresh chives
1 teaspoon lemon zest

1. Combine the Worcestershire sauce, lemon juice, broth, and Dijon mustard in a bowl. Stir to mix well.
2. On a clean work surface, rub the pork chops with salt and ground black pepper.
3. Heat the olive oil in a nonstick skillet over medium-high heat until shimmering.
4. Add the pork chops and sear for 16 minutes or until well browned. Flip the pork halfway through the cooking time. Transfer to a plate and set aside.
5. Pour the sauce mixture in the skillet and cook for 2 minutes or until warmed through and lightly thickened. Mix in the chives and lemon zest.
6. Baste the pork with the sauce mixture and serve immediately.

Pork Souvlakia with Tzatziki Sauce

Prep time: 20 minutes | Cook time: 12 minutes | Serves 4

¼ cup lemon juice
1 tablespoon dried oregano
¼ teaspoon salt
¼ teaspoon ground black pepper

1 pound (454 g) pork tenderloin, cut into 1-inch cubes
1 tablespoon olive oil

Tzatziki Sauce:
½ cup plain Greek yogurt
1 large cucumber, peeled, deseeded and grated
1 tablespoon fresh lemon juice

4 cloves garlic, minced or grated
¼ teaspoon ground black pepper

Special Equipment:
8 bamboo skewers, soaked in water for at least 30 minutes

1. Combine the lemon juice, oregano, salt, and ground black pepper in a large bowl. Stir to mix well.
2. Dunk the pork cubes in the bowl of mixture, then toss to coat well. Wrap the bowl in plastic and refrigerate to marinate for 10 minutes or overnight.
3. Preheat the oven to 450ºF (235ºC) or broil. Grease a baking sheet with the olive oil.
4. Remove the bowl from the refrigerator. Run the bamboo skewers through the pork cubes. Set the skewers on the baking sheet, then brush with marinade.
5. Broil the skewers in the preheated oven for 12 minutes or until well browned. Flip skewers at least 3 times during the broiling.
6. Meanwhile, combine the ingredients for the tzatziki sauce in a small bowl.
7. Remove the skewers from the oven and baste with the tzatziki sauce and serve immediately.

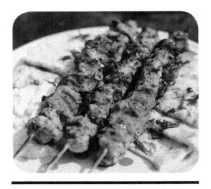

Tips: You can serve the pork souvlakia and tzatziki sauce in the pocket of pita breads. And you can replace the pork cubes with lamb meat or beef meat for a distinct flavor.

Per Serving
calories: 260 | fat: 7.0g
protein: 28.0g | carbs: 21.0g
fiber: 3.0g | sugar: 3.0g
sodium: 360mg

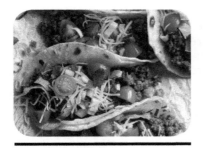

Tip: To make this a complete meal, you can serve it with roasted Brussels sprouts or broccoli and kale soup.

Per Serving
calories: 295 | fat: 6.0g
protein: 19.0g | carbs: 43.0g
fiber: 6.0g | sugar: 3.0g
sodium: 600mg

Beef, Tomato, and Pepper Tortillas

Prep time: 15 minutes | Cook time: 0 minutes | Serves 6

6 whole wheat flour tortillas (10-inch)
6 large romaine lettuce leaves
12 ounces (340 g) cooked deli roast beef, thinly sliced
1 cup diced red bell peppers

1 cup diced tomatoes
1 tablespoon red wine vinegar
1 teaspoon cumin
¼ teaspoon freshly ground black pepper
1 tablespoon olive oil

1. Unfold the tortillas on a clean work surface, then top each tortilla with a lettuce leaf. Divide the roast beef over the leaf.
2. Combine the remaining ingredients in a bowl. Stir to mix well. Pour the mixture over the beef.
3. Fold the tortillas over the fillings, then roll them up. Serve immediately.

Classic Stroganoff

Prep time: 15 minutes | Cook time: 20 minutes | Serves 5

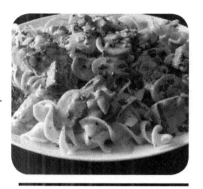

5 ounces (142 g) cooked egg noodles
2 teaspoons olive oil
1 pound (454 g) beef tenderloin tips, boneless, sliced into 2-inch strips
1½ cups white button mushrooms, sliced
½ cup onion, minced

1 tablespoon all-purpose flour
½ cup dry white wine
1 (14.5-ounce / 411-g) can fat-free, low-sodium beef broth
1 teaspoon Dijon mustard
½ cup fat-free sour cream
¼ teaspoon salt
¼ teaspoon black pepper

1. Put the cooked egg noodles on a large plate.
2. Heat the olive oil in a nonstick skillet over high heat until shimmering.
3. Add the beef and sauté for 3 minutes or until lightly browned. Remove the beef from the skillet and set on the plate with noodles.
4. Add the mushrooms and onion to the skillet and sauté for 5 minutes or until tender and the onion browns.
5. Add the flour and cook for a minute. Add the white wine and cook for 2 more minutes.
6. Add the beef broth and Dijon mustard. Bring to a boil. Keep stirring. Reduce the heat to low and simmer for another 5 minutes.
7. Add the beef back to the skillet and simmer for an additional 3 minutes. Add the remaining ingredients and simmer for 1 minute.
8. Pour them over the egg noodles and beef, and serve immediately.

Tip: How to cook the egg noodles:
Bring a pot of water to a boil, then add the noodles and cook for 1 minute or until al dente. Rinse the noodles in cold water and pat dry before using.

Per Serving
calories: 275 | fat: 7.0g
protein: 23.0g | carbs: 29.0g | fiber: 4.0g
sugar: 3.0g | sodium: 250mg

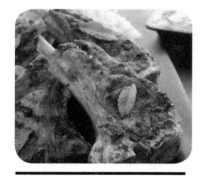

Tip: If you are fancy of the spicy taste of the lamb cutlets, you can sprinkle the cooked cutlets with chipotle chili powder or red pepper flakes before serving.

Per Serving
calories: 297 | fat: 18.8g
protein: 31.0g | carbs: 1.0g
fiber: 0g | sugar: 0g
sodium: 100mg

Easy Lime Lamb Cutlets

Prep time: 4 hours 20 minutes | Cook time: 8 minutes
Serves 4

¼ cup freshly squeezed lime juice
2 tablespoons lime zest
2 tablespoons chopped fresh parsley
Sea salt and freshly ground

black pepper, to taste
1 tablespoon extra-virgin olive oil
12 lamb cutlets (about 1½ pounds / 680 g in total)

1. Combine the lime juice and zest, parsley, salt, black pepper, and olive oil in a large bowl. Stir to mix well.
2. Dunk the lamb cutlets in the bowl of the lime mixture, then toss to coat well. Wrap the bowl in plastic and refrigerate to marinate for at least 4 hours.
3. Preheat the oven to 450ºF (235ºC) or broil. Line a baking sheet with aluminum foil.
4. Remove the bowl from the refrigerator and let sit for 10 minutes, then discard the marinade. Arrange the lamb cutlets on the baking sheet.
5. Broil the lamb in the preheated oven for 8 minutes or until it reaches your desired doneness. Flip the cutlets with tongs to make sure they are cooked evenly.
6. Serve immediately.

Spinach, Pear, and Walnut Salad

Prep time: 10 minutes | Cook time: 0 minutes
Serves 2

2 tablespoons apple cider
vinegar
1 teaspoon peeled and
grated fresh ginger
½ teaspoon Dijon mustard
2 tablespoons extra-virgin

olive oil
½ teaspoon sea salt
4 cups baby spinach
½ pear, cored, peeled, and
chopped
¼ cup chopped walnuts

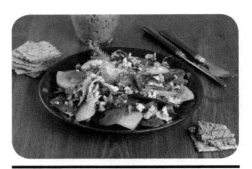

1. Combine the vinegar, ginger, mustard, olive oil, and salt in a small bowl. Stir to mix well.
2. Combine the remaining ingredients in a large serving bowl, then toss to combine well.
3. Pour the vinegar dressing in the bowl of salad and toss before serving.

Tip: You can replace the pear with the same amount of chopped apples, strawberries, or blueberries for different flours.

Per Serving
calories: 229 | fat: 20.4g
protein: 3.5g | carbs: 10.7g
fiber: 3.4g | sugar: 4.9g
sodium: 644mg

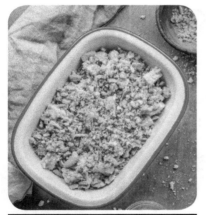

Tips: You can use the whole-wheat pastry flour to replace the all-purpose flour. And you can use the green beans to replace the peas.

Per Serving
calories: 250 | fat: 7.0g
protein: 25.0g | carbs: 24.0g
fiber: 3.0g | sugar: 5.0g
sodium: 290mg

Ritzy Beef Stew

Prep time: 20 minutes | Cook time: 2 hours | Serves 6

2 tablespoons all-purpose flour
1 tablespoon Italian seasoning
2 pounds (907 g) top round,
cut into ¾-inch cubes
2 tablespoons olive oil
4 cups low-sodium chicken
broth, divided
1½ pounds (680 g) cremini
mushrooms, rinsed, stems
removed, and quartered
1 large onion, coarsely

chopped
3 cloves garlic, minced
3 medium carrots, peeled and
cut into ½-inch pieces
1 cup frozen peas
1 tablespoon fresh thyme,
minced
1 tablespoon red wine vinegar
½ teaspoon freshly ground
black pepper

1. Combine the flour and Italian seasoning in a large bowl. Dredge the beef cubes in the bowl to coat well.
2. Heat the olive oil in a pot over medium heat until shimmering.
3. Add the beef to the single layer in the pot and cook for 2 to 4 minutes or until golden brown on all sides. Flip the beef cubes frequently.
4. Remove the beef from the pot and set aside, then add ¼ cup of chicken broth to the pot.
5. Add the mushrooms and sauté for 4 minutes or until soft. Remove the mushrooms from the pot and set aside.
6. Pour ¼ cup of chicken broth in the pot. Add the onions and garlic to the pot and sauté for 4 minutes or until translucent.
7. Put the beef back to the pot and pour in the remaining broth. Bring to a boil.
8. Reduce the heat to low and cover. Simmer for 45 minutes. Stir periodically.
9. Add the carrots, mushroom, peas, and thyme to the pot and simmer for 45 more minutes or until the vegetables are soft.
10. Open the lid, drizzle with red wine vinegar and season with black pepper. Stir and serve in a large bowl.

Slow Cooked Beef and Vegetables Roast

Prep time: 15 minutes | Cook time: 4 hours | Serves 4

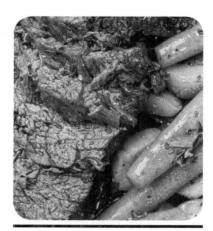

1 tablespoon olive oil
2 medium celery stalks, halved lengthwise and cut into 3-inch pieces
4 medium carrots, scrubbed, halved lengthwise, and cut into 3-inch pieces
1 medium onion, cut in eighths
1¼ pounds (567 g) lean chuck roast, boneless, trimmed of fat
2 teaspoons Worcestershire sauce
1 tablespoon balsamic vinegar
2 tablespoons water
1 tablespoon onion soup mix
½ teaspoon ground black pepper

1. Grease a slow cooker with olive oil.
2. Put the celery, carrots, and onion in the slow cooker, then add the beef.
3. Top them with Worcestershire sauce, balsamic vinegar, and water, then sprinkle with onion soup mix and black pepper.
4. Cover and cook on high for 4 hours.
5. Allow to cool for 20 minutes, then serve them on a large plate.

Tip: If you don't have the onion soup mix, you can replace it with the same amount of grated onion, garlic powder, and salt mix.

Per Serving
calories: 250 | fat: 6.0g
protein: 33.0g | carbs: 15.0g
fiber: 3.0g | sugar: 6.0g
sodium: 510mg

Chapter 13 Soups, Salads, and Sandwiches

Chicken and Zoodle Soup

Prep time: 10 minutes | Cook time: 15 minutes | Serves 4

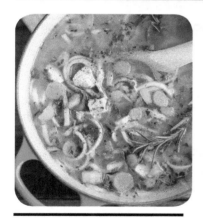

Tip: To make this a complete meal, you can serve it with beef steak or seared pork chops.

Per Serving
calories: 292 | fat: 16.9g
protein: 25.8g | carbs: 10.8g
fiber: 1.6g | sugar: 3.2g
sodium: 772mg

2 tablespoons extra-virgin olive oil
12 ounces (340 g) chicken breast, cut into bite-sized pieces
2 carrots, chopped
2 celery stalks, chopped
1 onion, chopped
2 garlic cloves
1 teaspoon dried thyme
6 cups low-sodium chicken broth
1 teaspoon sea salt
2 medium zucchinis, spiralized

1. Heat the olive oil in a pot over medium-high heat until shimmering.
2. Add the chicken and sear for 5 minutes or until well browned. Remove the cooked chicken from the pot and set aside on a plate.
3. Add the carrots, celery, and onion to the pot and sauté for 5 minutes or until tender.
4. Add the garlic and sauté for 1 minutes or until fragrant.
5. Add the thyme, chicken broth, and salt. Bring to a boil, then reduce the heat to medium.
6. Put the chicken back to the pot and add the spiralized zucchini. Simmer for 2 minutes or until the zucchini is tender. Keep stirring during the simmering.
7. Pour the soup in a large bowl and serve immediately.

Ritzy Calabaza Squash Soup

Prep time: 15 minutes | Cook time: 45 minutes | Serves 8

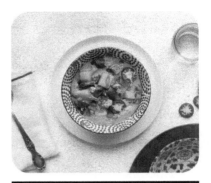

2 pounds (907 g) calabaza squash, peeled and chopped
1 large tomato, chopped
1 medium onion, chopped
1 medium green bell pepper, chopped
1 scotch bonnet chili, deseeded and minced
8 scallions, chopped
3 sprigs fresh thyme
1 tablespoon minced ginger root
8 cups low-sodium vegetable broth
Juice of 1 lime
¼ cup chopped cilantro
Salt, to taste
¼ cup toasted pepitas

1. Put the calabaza squash, tomato, onion, bell pepper, scotch bonnet, scallions, thyme, and ginger roots in a saucepan, then pour in the vegetable broth.
2. Bring to a boil over medium-high heat. Reduce the heat to low, then simmer for 45 minutes or until the vegetables are soft. Stir constantly.
3. Add the lime juice, cilantro, and salt. Pour the soup in a large bowl, then discard the thyme sprigs and garnish with pepitas before serving.

Tip: You can use 1 teaspoon of dried fresh thyme to replace the fresh thyme sprigs.
If you can't find the scotch bonnet chili, you can use jalapeño pepper to replace it.

Per Serving
calories: 50 | fat: 0g
protein: 2.0g | carbs: 12.0g
fiber: 4.0g | sugar: 5.0g
sodium: 20mg

Simple Buttercup Squash Soup

Prep time: 15 minutes | Cook time: 33 minutes | Serves 6

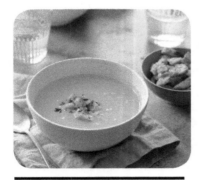

2 tablespoons extra-virgin olive oil
1 medium onion, chopped
1½ pounds (680 g) buttercup squash, peeled, deseeded, and cut into 1-inch chunks
4 cups vegetable broth
½ teaspoon kosher salt
¼ teaspoon ground white pepper
Ground nutmeg, to taste

1. Heat the olive oil in a pot over medium-high heat until shimmering.
2. Add the onion and sauté for 3 minutes or until translucent.
3. Add the buttercup squash, vegetable broth, salt, and pepper. Stir to mix well. Bring to a boil.
4. Reduce the heat to low and simmer for 30 minutes or until the buttercup squash is soft.
5. Pour the soup in a food processor, then pulse to purée until creamy and smooth.
6. Pour the soup in a large serving bowl, then sprinkle with ground nutmeg and serve.

Tips: You can use the same amount of butternut squash to replace the buttercup squash if you really cannot find one.
You can use the same amount of chicken bone broth to replace the vegetable broth.

Per Serving (1¹/₃ Cups)
calories: 110 | fat: 5.0g
protein: 1.0g | carbs: 18.0g
fiber: 4.0g | sugar: 4.0g
sodium: 166mg

Turkey, Barley and Vegetable Stock

Prep time: 25 minutes | Cook time: 3 hours 7 minutes
Serves 8

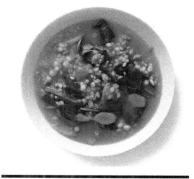

2 tablespoons avocado oil
1 pound (454 g) ground turkey
28 ounces (1.3 kg) tomatoes, diced
2 tablespoons sugar-free tomato paste
4 cups low-sodium chicken broth
1 (15-ounce / 425-g) package frozen peppers and onions (about 2½ cups)
1 (15-ounce / 425-g) package frozen chopped carrots (about 2½ cups)
¹⁄₃ cup dry barley
2 bay leaves
1 teaspoon kosher salt
¼ teaspoon freshly ground black pepper

1. Heat the avocado oil in a pot over medium-high heat.
2. Add the turkey and sauté for 7 minutes or until lightly browned.
3. Add the tomatoes, tomato paste, and chicken broth. Stir to mix well.
4. Add the peppers and onions, carrots, barley, bay leaves, salt, and pepper. Stir to mix well.
5. Bring to a boil. Reduce the heat to low, then cover the pot and simmer for 3 hours.
6. Once the simmering is finished, allow to cool for 20 minutes, then discard the bay leaves and pour the soup in a large bowl to serve.

Tip: You can also use ground chicken to replace the ground turkey.
Fresh carrots, onions, and peppers work better than the frozen ones, so if you choose the fresh ones, you can sauté then with turkey.

Per Serving (1¼ Cups)
calories: 253 | fat: 12.0g
protein: 19.0g | carbs: 21.0g
fiber: 7.0g | sugar: 7.0g
sodium: 560mg

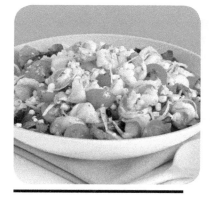

Tip: You can use Mexican queso fresco or cotija to replace the feta cheese.

Per Serving
calories: 195 | fat: 10.0g
protein: 17.0g | carbs: 12.0g
fiber: 4.0g | sugar: 3.0g
sodium: 440mg

Shrimp and Cherry Tomato Salad

Prep time: 20 minutes | Cook time: 4 minutes | Serves 8

2 tablespoons extra virgin olive oil, divided
1 pound (454 g) large shrimps, peeled and deveined
2 avocados, peeled and cubed
2 ears fresh corn, kernels sliced off
2 cups cherry tomatoes, halved
3 ounces (85 g) reduced-fat
feta cheese, cubed
1 tablespoon balsamic vinegar
¼ teaspoon cumin
¼ teaspoon celery seeds
¼ cup slivered fresh basil
1 tablespoon fresh lemon juice
⅛ teaspoon salt
¼ teaspoon freshly ground black pepper

1. Heat 1 tablespoon of olive oil in a nonstick skillet over medium heat until shimmering.
2. Add the shrimps and grill for 4 minutes or until opaque. Flip the shrimps halfway through the cooking time.
3. Combine the remaining ingredients in a large salad bowl, then add the shrimps and toss to combine well.
4. Serve immediately.

Citrus Pork Tenderloin

Prep time: 10 minutes | Cook time: 30 minutes | Serves 4

¼ cup freshly squeezed orange juice
2 teaspoons orange zest
1 teaspoon low-sodium soy sauce
1 teaspoon honey
1 teaspoon grated fresh ginger
2 teaspoons minced garlic
1½ pounds (680 g) pork tenderloin roast, fat trimmed
1 tablespoon extra-virgin olive oil

1. Combine the orange juice and zest, soy sauce, honey, ginger, and garlic in a large bowl. Stir to mix well. Dunk the pork in the bowl and press to coat well.
2. Wrap the bowl in plastic and refrigerate to marinate for at least 2 hours.
3. Preheat the oven to 400ºF (205ºC).
4. Remove the bowl from the refrigerator and discard the marinade.
5. Heat the olive oil in an oven-safe skillet over medium-high heat until shimmering.
6. Add the pork and sear for 5 minutes. Flip the pork halfway through the cooking time.
7. Arrange the skillet in the preheated oven and roast the pork for 25 minutes or until well browned. Flip the pork halfway through the cooking time.
8. Transfer the pork on a plate. Allow to cool before serving.

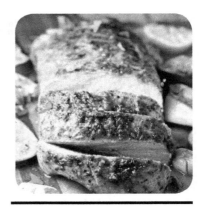

Tip: You can slice the pork tenderloin and wrap it with cucumber and pepper slices in tortillas to serve.

Per Serving
calories: 228 | fat: 9.0g
protein: 34.0g | carbs: 4.0g
fiber: 0g | sugar: 3.0g
sodium: 486mg

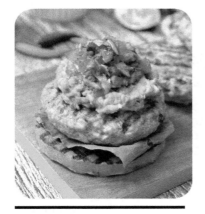

Mexican Turkey Sliders

Prep time: 15 minutes | Cook time: 6 minutes | Serves 7

1 pound (454 g) lean ground turkey
1 tablespoon chili powder
½ teaspoon garlic powder
¼ teaspoon ground black pepper
7 mini whole-wheat hamburger buns
7 tomato slices
3½ slices reduced-fat pepper Jack cheese, cut in half
½ mashed avocado

1. Preheat the grill to high heat.
2. Combine the ground turkey, chili powder, garlic powder, and black pepper in a large bow. Stir to mix well.
3. Divide and shape the mixture into 7 patties, then arrange the patties on the preheated grill grates.
4. Grill for 6 minutes or until well browned. Flip the patties halfway through.
5. Assemble the patties with buns, tomato slices, cheese slices, and mashed avocado to make the sliders, then serve immediately.

Tip: You can use gluten-free bread to replace the hamburger buns.

Per Serving
calories: 225 | fat: 9.0g
protein: 17.0g | carbs: 21.0g
fiber: 4.0g | sugar: 6.0g
sodium: 230mg

Cheesy Vegetable and Hummus Pitas

Prep time: 15 minutes | Cook time: 0 minutes
Serves 4

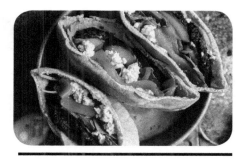

4 whole wheat pitas, sliced into pockets
2 tablespoons light mayonnaise
½ cup hummus
2¼ ounces (64 g) reduced-fat Swiss cheese, cut into 4 slices

¼ cup sunflower seeds
1 large tomato, cut into 4 equal slices
1 medium cucumber, sliced
1 medium red onion, thinly sliced
4 romaine lettuce leaves

Tip: To make this a complete meal, you can serve it with chicken chunks, spinach, and kale salad.

1. Smear the insides of the pita pockets with mayo.
2. Divide the hummus on each cheese slice and smear to spread evenly, then sprinkle with sunflower seeds.
3. Sit the tomato slices, cucumber slices, onion slices, and lettuce leaves on top of the hummus alternatively.
4. Then stuff the pitas with these slices and serve immediately.

Per Serving
calories: 170 | fat: 6.0g
protein: 8.0g | carbs: 23.0g
fiber: 4.0g | sugar: 7.0g
sodium: 280mg

Seafood, Mango, and Avocado Salad

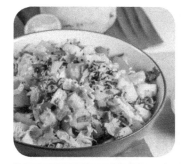

Prep time: 30 minutes | Cook time: 20 minutes | Serves 4

1 cup quinoa, rinsed
½ pound (227 g) medium shrimps, peeled and deveined
½ pound (227 g) scallops
1 tablespoon olive oil
½ red bell pepper, chopped
1 roma plum tomatoes, deseeded and chopped

1 jalapeño pepper, stemmed and finely chopped
½ cup cooked black beans
1 mango, chopped
1 avocado, chopped
2 small scallions, chopped
2 tablespoons cilantro leaves, chopped

Tip: You can use the same amount of cooked edamame to replace the black beans.

Citrus Dressing:
2 tablespoons lime juice
2 tablespoons orange juice
1 teaspoon honey

¼ teaspoon cayenne pepper
1 tablespoon extra virgin olive oil
Sea salt, to taste

Per Serving
calories: 470 | fat: 16.0g
protein: 30.0g | carbs: 56.0g | fiber: 10.0g
sugar: 16.0g
sodium: 320mg

1. Pour the quinoa in a pot, then pour in enough water to cover. Bring to a boil, then reduce the heat to low and simmer to 10 to 15 minutes or until the liquid has been absorbed. Fluffy with a fork and let stand until ready to use.
2. Meanwhile, combine the ingredients for the citrus dressing in a small bowl. Stir to mix well. Set aside until ready to use.
3. Put the shrimps and scallops in a separate bowl, then drizzle with the olive oil. Toss to coat well.
4. Add the oiled shrimps and scallops in a nonstick skillet and grill over medium-high heat for 4 minutes or until opaque. Flip them halfway through. Remove them from the skillet and allow to cool.
5. Combine the cooked quinoa, shrimp and scallops with bell pepper, tomato, jalapeño, beans, mango, avocado, and scallions in a large salad bowl, then drizzle with the citrus dressing. Toss to combine well.
6. Garnish with cilantro leaves and serve immediately.

Crispy Apple Chips

Prep time: 10 minutes | Cook time: 2 hours | Serves 4

2 medium apples, sliced
1 teaspoon ground cinnamon

1. Preheat the oven to 200ºF (93ºC). Line a baking sheet with parchment paper.
2. Arrange the apple slices on the prepared baking sheet, then sprinkle with cinnamon.
3. Bake in the preheated oven for 2 hours or until crispy. Flip the apple chips halfway through the cooking time.
4. Allow to cool for 10 minutes and serve warm.

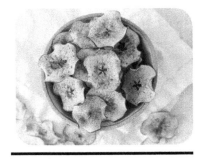

Per Serving
calories: 50 | fat: 0g
protein: 0g | carbs: 13.0g
fiber: 2.0g | sugar: 9.0g
sodium: 0mg

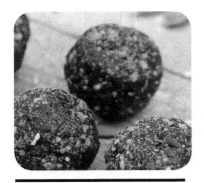

Tip: For a distinct twist, you can roll the date balls in the coconut flakes and dust them with some honey before serving.

Per Serving (1 Ball)
calories: 113 | fat: 7.1g
protein: 2.9g | carbs: 12.0g
fiber: 2.0g | sugar: 7.8g
sodium: 10mg

Date and Almond Balls with Seeds

Prep time: 15 minutes | Cook time: 0 minutes
Serves 36 Balls

1 pound (454 g) pitted dates
½ pound (227 g) blanched almonds
¼ cup water
¼ cup butter, at room temperature

1 teaspoon ground cardamom
1 teaspoon vanilla extract
½ teaspoon ground cinnamon
2 tablespoons ground flaxseed
1 cup toasted sesame seeds

1. In a food processor, add the pitted dates, almonds, water, butter, cardamon, vanilla, and cinnamon, and pulse until the mixture has broken down into a smooth paste.
2. Scoop out the paste and form into 36 equal-sized balls with your hands.
3. Spread out the flaxseed and sesame seeds on a baking sheet. Roll the balls in the seed mixture until they are evenly coated on all sides.
4. Serve immediately or store in an airtight container in the fridge for 2 days.

Apple Cinnamon Chimichanga

Prep time: 15 minutes | Cook time: 15 minutes
Serves 4

2 apple, cored and chopped
3 tablespoons splenda, divided
¼ cup water

½ teaspoon ground cinnamon
4 (8-inch) whole-wheat flour tortillas
Nonstick cooking spray

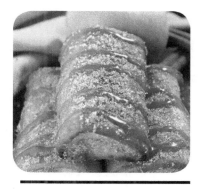

Special Equipment:
4 toothpicks, soaked in water for at least 30 minutes

1. Preheat the oven to 400ºF (205ºC). Line a baking sheet with parchment paper and set aside.
2. Make the apple filling: Add the apples, 2 tablespoons of splenda, water, and cinnamon to a medium saucepan over medium heat. Stir to combine and allow the mixture to boil for 5 minutes, or until the apples are fork-tender, but not mushy.
3. Remove the apple filling from the heat and let it cool to room temperature.
4. Make the chimichangas: Place the tortillas on a lightly floured surface.
5. Spoon 2 teaspoons of prepared apple filling onto each tortilla and fold the tortilla over to enclose the filling. Roll each tortilla up and run the toothpicks through to secure. Spritz the tortillas lightly with nonstick cooking spray.
6. Arrange the tortillas on the prepared baking sheet, seam-side down. Scatter the remaining splenda all over the tortillas.
7. Bake in the preheated oven for 10 minutes, flipping the tortillas halfway through, or until they are crispy and golden brown on each side.
8. Remove from the oven to four plates and serve while warm.

Tip: You can garnish the chimichangas with a dollop of whipped cream or a scoop of ice cream before serving.

Per Serving (1 Chimichanga)
calories: 201 | fat: 6.2g
protein: 3.9g | carbs: 32.8g
fiber: 5.0g | sugar: 7.9g
sodium: 241mg

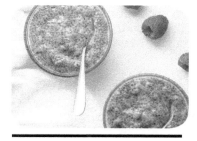

Tip: The chia and raspberry seed pudding can be made the night before serving. Just allow the pudding to refrigerate overnight.

Per Serving
calories: 122 | fat: 5.2g
protein: 3.1g | carbs: 17.9g
fiber: 9.0g | sugar: 6.8g
sodium: 51mg

Chia and Raspberry Pudding

Prep time: 1 hours | Cook time: 0 minutes | Serves 4

1 cup unsweetened vanilla almond milk
2 cup plus ½ cup raspberries, divided

¼ cup chia seeds
1½ teaspoons lemon juice
½ teaspoon lemon zest
1 tablespoon honey

1. Stir together the almond milk, 2 cups of raspberries, chia seeds, lemon juice, lemon zest, and honey in a small bowl.
2. Transfer the bowl to the fridge to thicken for at least 1 hour, or until a pudding-like texture is achieved.
3. When the pudding is ready, give it a good stir. Scatter with the remaining ½ cup raspberries and serve immediately.

Easy Banana Mug Cake

Prep time: 10 minutes | Cook time: 1 minutes | Serves 1

½ ripe banana, mashed
3 tablespoons egg white
1 teaspoon oat flour
½ tablespoon vanilla protein powder
1 teaspoon rolled oats
1 teaspoon cocoa powder
½ teaspoon baking powder
2 tablespoons stevia
1 teaspoon olive oil
2 teaspoons chopped walnuts

1. Whisk together the banana and egg whites in a bowl.
2. Add the flour, vanilla protein powder, rolled oats, cocoa powder, baking powder, and stevia to the bowl. Stir to mix well.
3. Grease a microwave-safe mug with olive oil.
4. Pour the mixture in the bowl, then scatter with chopped walnuts.
5. Microwave them for 1 minutes or until puffed.
6. Serve immediately.

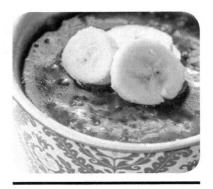

Tip: You can replace the banana with other fruits to try out a different taste of the mug cake, such as mashed apple or crushed berries.

Per Serving
calories: 211 | fat: 12.0g
protein: 11.3g | carbs: 46.7g
fiber: 2.8g | sugar: 6.6g
sodium: 97mg

Pumpkin and Raspberry Muffins

Prep time: 20 minutes | Cook time: 25 minutes
Serves 12 Muffins

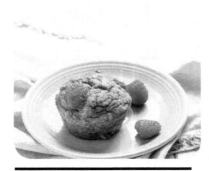

Tip: You can use the almond flour or arrowroot flour to replace the coconut flour.

Per Serving (1 Muffin)
calories: 223 | fat: 15.6g
protein: 4.4g | carbs: 29.3g
fiber: 2.9g | sugar: 7.7g
sodium: 76mg

¾ cup blanched almond flour
½ cup coconut flour
3 tablespoons tapioca
1 tablespoon cinnamon
1 tablespoon baking powder
Pinch of nutmeg
½ cup stevia in raw
¼ teaspoon salt
1 cup puréed pumpkin
4 large eggs, whites and yolks separated
1½ teaspoons vanilla extract
½ cup coconut oil
10 drops liquid stevia
1½ cups frozen raspberries

1. Preheat the oven to 350ºF (180ºC). Line a 12-cup muffin pan with paper muffin cups.
2. Combine the flours, tapioca, cinnamon, baking powder, nutmeg, stevia in raw, and salt in a large bowl. Stir to mix well.
3. Mix in the puréed pumpkin, egg yolks, vanilla extract, coconut oil, and liquid stevia until a batter forms. Divide the batter into the muffin cups.
4. Whip the egg whites in a separate large bowl until it forms the stiff peaks.
5. Top the batter with the beaten egg whites and raspberries.
6. Place the muffin pan in the preheated oven and bake for 25 minutes or until a toothpick inserted in the center of the muffins comes out clean.
7. Remove the muffins from the oven and allow to cool for 5 minutes before serving.

Avocado Cilantro Dressing

Prep time: 5 minutes | Cook time: 0 minutes | Makes 1 cup

1 large avocado, peeled and pitted
½ cup plain Greek yogurt
¾ cup fresh cilantro
1 tablespoon water
2 teaspoons freshly squeezed lime juice
⅛ teaspoon garlic powder
Pinch salt

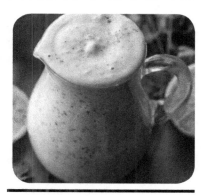

1. Process the avocado, yogurt, cilantro, water, lime juice, garlic powder, and salt in a blender until creamy and emulsified.
2. Chill for at least 30 minutes in the refrigerator to let the flavors blend.

Tips: If you prefer a thinner dressing, you can add a few tablespoons of water. It perfectly goes well with the cooked vegetables or tortilla chips, and it is a perfect substitute for mayo in a chicken salad.

Per Serving (¼ Cup)
calories: 92 | fat: 6.8g
protein: 4.1g | carbs: 4.9g
fiber: 2.3g | sugar: 1.0g
sodium: 52mg

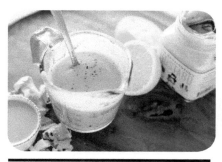

Tips: You can find the tahini that is made from sesame seeds in large supermarkets in the Middle Eastern section. It perfectly goes well with chicken and salads.

Per Serving (2 Tablespoons)
calories: 168 | fat: 13.1g
protein: 4.7g | carbs: 10.3g
fiber: 2.8g | sugar: 8.0g
sodium: 148mg

Lemon Tahini Dressing with Honey

Prep time: 5 minutes | Cook time: 0 minutes
Makes 1 cup

½ cup water
¾ cup unsalted tahini
⅓ cup freshly squeezed lemon juice
3 tablespoons honey
½ teaspoon salt

1. Mix together the water, tahini, lemon juice, honey, and salt in a medium bowl, and stir vigorously until well incorporated.
2. Store the leftover dressing in an airtight container in the fridge for up to 2 weeks and shake before using.

Red Pepper and Chickpea Spread

Prep time: 5 minutes | Cook time: 0 minutes
Makes 1¼ cups

1 (16-ounce / 454-g) jar roasted red bell peppers
1 cup canned low-sodium chickpeas, drained and rinsed
½ small jalapeño pepper, deseeded and stemmed
2 tablespoons water
2 tablespoons extra-virgin olive oil
1 to 2 teaspoons freshly squeezed lime juice
¼ teaspoon garlic powder
½ teaspoon salt
¼ teaspoon ground cumin
⅛ teaspoon freshly ground black pepper

1. In a food processor, add the bell peppers, chickpeas, jalapeño pepper, water, oil, lime juice, garlic powder, salt, cumin, and black pepper, and pulse until the mixture has a spreadable consistency.
2. Transfer to an airtight container and store in the fridge for up to 1 week.

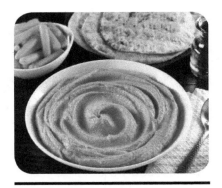

Tips: For a unique twist, you can add 2 to 3 tablespoons of unsalted tahini to this spread. You can serve it over the avocado toast or eggs.

Per Serving (2 Tablespoons)
calories: 52 | fat: 2.8g
protein: 1.1g | carbs: 4.7g
fiber: 2.2g | sugar: 2.0g
sodium: 138mg

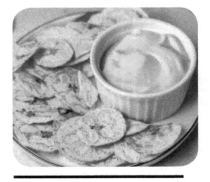

Tips: For a rich flavor, you can try adding ½ teaspoon freshly ground black pepper. It can be served as a dipping sauce or over the cooked shrimp.

Per Serving (2 Tablespoons)
calories: 43 | fat: 2.7g
protein: 0g | carbs: 2.7g
fiber: 0g | sugar: 1.1g
sodium: 168mg

Mayo Ketchup Sauce

Prep time: 5 minutes | Cook time: 0 minutes | Makes 1 cup

½ cup low-fat mayonnaise
6 tablespoons no-salt-added, no-sugar-added ketchup
1 teaspoon garlic powder

1. Whisk together the mayo, ketchup, and garlic powder in a small bowl until completely mixed.
2. You can store it in an airtight container in the fridge for up to 2 weeks.

Spicy Asian Dipping Sauce

Prep time: 5 minutes | Cook time: 0 minutes
Makes ½ cup

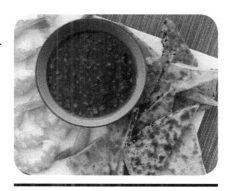

⅓ cup low-fat mayonnaise
1 to 2 teaspoons hot sauce, to your liking
2 teaspoons rice vinegar
1 teaspoon sesame oil

1. Stir together the mayo, hot sauce, rice vinegar, and oil in a small bowl until thoroughly smooth.
2. Chill for at least 30 minutes to blend the flavors.

Tips: For added spicy, you can increase the amount of hot sauce. You can serve the chicken lettuce wraps with this sauce on the side.

Per Serving (2 Tablespoons)
calories: 54 | fat: 4.7g
protein: 0g | carbs: 1.7g
fiber: 0g | sugar: 1.0g
sodium: 190mg

Easy Thai Peanut Sauce

Prep time: 10 minutes | Cook time: 0 minutes
Makes ⅔ cup

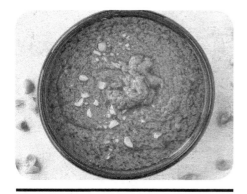

½ cup natural peanut butter
2 tablespoons rice vinegar
4 teaspoons sesame oil
2 to 4 teaspoons freshly squeezed lime juice, to your liking
2 to 2½ teaspoons hot sauce (optional)
1 teaspoon low-sodium soy sauce
1 teaspoon chopped peeled fresh ginger
1 teaspoon honey

1. Mix together the peanut butter, rice vinegar, sesame oil, lime juice, hot sauce (if desired), soy sauce, ginger, and honey in a small bowl, and whisk to combine well.
2. You can store it in an airtight container in the fridge for up to 2 weeks.

Tips: If the fresh ginger isn't available, you can use a pinch of ground ginger instead. Feel free to add more water if you like a thinner consistency.

Per Serving (2½ Tablespoons)
calories: 206 | fat: 16.7g
protein: 7.9g | carbs: 8.2g
fiber: 3.1g | sugar: 3.0g
sodium: 113mg

Chimichurri

Prep time: 5 minutes | Cook time: 0 minutes | Serves 4

½ cup Italian parsley
¼ cup extra-virgin olive oil
¼ cup fresh cilantro, stems removed
Zest of 1 lemon
2 tablespoons red wine vinegar
½ teaspoon sea salt
1 garlic clove, minced
¼ teaspoon red pepper flakes

1. Process all the ingredients in a food processor until smooth.
2. Store in an airtight container in the fridge for up to 2 days or in the freezer for 6 months.

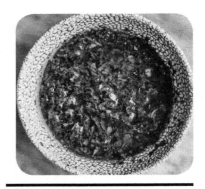

Tips: You can substitute half a jalapeño (deseeded and chopped) for the red pepper flakes. It tastes great paired with grilled steaks, or it can be used as a marinade for vegetables, pork, or chicken.

Per Serving
calories: 124 | fat: 13.7g
protein: 0g | carbs: 0.8g
fiber: 0g | sugar: 0.5g
sodium: 150mg

Appendix 1: Measurement conversion Chart

VOLUME EQUIVALENTS(DRY)

US STANDARD	METRIC (APPROXIMATE)
1/8 teaspoon	0.5 mL
1/4 teaspoon	1 mL
1/2 teaspoon	2 mL
3/4 teaspoon	4 mL
1 teaspoon	5 mL
1 tablespoon	15 mL
1/4 cup	59 mL
1/2 cup	118 mL
3/4 cup	177 mL
1 cup	235 mL
2 cups	475 mL
3 cups	700 mL
4 cups	1 L

VOLUME EQUIVALENTS(LIQUID)

US STANDARD	US STANDARD (OUNCES)	METRIC (APPROXIMATE)
2 tablespoons	1 fl.oz.	30 mL
1/4 cup	2 fl.oz.	60 mL
1/2 cup	4 fl.oz.	120 mL
1 cup	8 fl.oz.	240 mL
1 1/2 cup	12 fl.oz.	355 mL
2 cups or 1 pint	16 fl.oz.	475 mL
4 cups or 1 quart	32 fl.oz.	1 L
1 gallon	128 fl.oz.	4 L

TEMPERATURES EQUIVALENTS

FAHRENHEIT(F)	CELSIUS(C) (APPROXIMATE)
225 °F	107 °C
250 °F	120 °C
275 °F	135 °C
300 °F	150 °C
325 °F	160 °C
350 °F	180 °C
375 °F	190 °C
400 °F	205 °C
425 °F	220 °C
450 °F	235 °C
475 °F	245 °C
500 °F	260 °C

WEIGHT EQUIVALENTS

US STANDARD	METRIC (APPROXIMATE)
1 ounce	28 g
2 ounces	57 g
5 ounces	142 g
10 ounces	284 g
15 ounces	425 g
16 ounces (1 pound)	455 g
1.5 pounds	680 g
2 pounds	907 g

Appendix 2: Recipes Index

A

Apple Cinnamon Chimichanga 63
Aromatic Toasted Pumpkin Seeds........... 20
Avocado Cilantro Dressing 65

B

Bacon-Wrapped Shrimps 21
Beef, Tomato, and Pepper Tortillas 54
Black Bean and Tomato Soup with Lime
Yogurt.. 36
Blackened Spatchcock with Lime Aioli...... 49
Broiled Teriyaki Salmon 40
Brown Rice with Carrot, and Scrambled Egg
.... 37
Brussels Sprout with Fried Eggs............. 15
Butter-Lemon Grilled Cod on Asparagus... 42
Butter-Orange Yams 26
Butternut Noodles With Mushroom Sauce.. 31

C

Carrot and Oat Pancakes 16
Cheesy Broccoli Bites 21
Cheesy Mushroom and Pesto Flatbreads .. 30
Cheesy Spinach and Egg Casserole 17
Cheesy Summer Squash and Quinoa
Casserole 33
Cheesy Vegetable and Hummus Pitas 61
Chia and Raspberry Pudding 63
Chicken and Zoodle Soup 57
Chimichurri...................................... 68
Chipotle Chili Pork 53
Cilantro Lime Shrimp 44
Cioppino (Seafood and Tomato Stew)...... 43
Citrus Chicken Thighs......................... 46
Citrus Pork Tenderloin 60
Classic Stroganoff............................. 55
Classic Texas Caviar........................... 36
Collard Greens with Tomato 32
Creamy and Aromatic Chicken............... 46
Creamy and Cheesy Chicken Chile Casserole
.... 47

Creamy Macaroni and Cheese 33
Crispy Apple Chips............................. 62
Crispy Cowboy Black Bean Fritters 34

D

Dandelion and Beet Greens 35
Date and Almond Balls with Seeds 62

E

Easy Banana Mug Cake 64
Easy Caprese Skewers 22
Easy Lime Lamb Cutlets 55
Easy Thai Peanut Sauce....................... 67
Easy Turkey Breakfast Patties................ 18

F

Fresh Rosemary Trout 42

G

Garlicky Mushrooms........................... 27
Grilled Shrimp Skewers with Yogurt 43
Grilled Tofu with Sesame Seeds............. 22

H

Herbed Chicken and Artichoke Hearts...... 45
Homemade Vegetable Chili 31

K

Kale Chips 23

L

Lemon Parsley White Fish Fillets 41
Lemon Tahini Dressing with Honey.......... 65
Lime Asparagus with Cashews................ 28

M

Macaroni and Vegetable Pie....................35
Marinated Grilled Salmon with Lemongrass ..
....39
Mayo Ketchup Sauce............................66
Black Bean, Corn, and Chicken Soup.......37
Mexican Turkey Sliders.........................60

P

Panko Coconut Shrimp..........................44
Peanut Butter and Berry Oatmeal..........19
Pecan-Oatmeal Pancakes......................19
Pork Diane...53
Pork Souvlakia with Tzatziki Sauce.........54
Pumpkin and Raspberry Muffins.............64

Q

Quick Breakfast Yogurt Sundae..............20

R

Red Kidney Beans with Tomatoes...........39
Red Pepper and Chickpea Spread...........66
Ritzy Beef Stew....................................56
Ritzy Calabaza Squash Soup..................58
Ritzy Jerked Chicken Breasts.................49
Roasted Asparagus and Red Peppers.......25
Roasted Brussels Sprouts with Wild Rice
Bowl...30
Roasted Chicken with Root Vegetables.....48
Roasted Delicata Squash with Thyme......24
Roasted Tomato and Bell Pepper Soup.....29
Roasted Tomato Brussels Sprouts...........26
Roasted Vegetable and Chicken Tortillas ..40

S

Sautéed Collard Greens and Cabbage......24
Sautéed Zucchini and Tomatoes.............29
Savory Breakfast Egg Bites....................16
Scrumptious Orange Muffins..................18
Sesame Bok Choy with Almonds.............28
Shrimp Coleslaw...................................45
Shrimp and Cherry Tomato Salad...........59
Simple Buttercup Squash Soup...............58
Simple Deviled Eggs.............................23
Simple Grain-Free Biscuits.....................15
Simple Sautéed Greens.........................27
Slow Cooked Beef and Vegetables Roast...57
Spaghetti Puttanesca............................34
Spicy Asian Dipping Sauce.....................67
Spinach, Pear, and Walnut Salad............56
Chicken with Carrot, and Kale...............51
Sumptuous Lamb and Pomegranate Salad52
Seafood, Mango, and Avocado Salad.......61

T

Tarragon Spring Peas............................25
Tartar Tuna Patties...............................41
Turkey Meatball and Vegetable Kabobs....50
Turkey, Barley and Vegetable Stock.........59

V

Vanilla Coconut Pancakes......................17

W

Wilted Dandelion Greens with Sweet Onion
....32
Wild Rice Cranberries Salad...................38

Lightning Source UK Ltd.
Milton Keynes UK
UKHW021436121021
392072UK00002B/76

9 781952 613821